Essential Lists for MRCP

Dr Stuart McPherson BSc MBChB MRCP
Senior House Officer in Infectious Diseases
North Glasgow University NHS Trust

Dr Duncan Fullerton MBChB DTM&H, MRCP (UK)
Specialist Registrar in Respiratory/General Medicine
Manchester Royal Infirmary

Dr James Greenwood MBChB
Senior House Officer in Medicine
Central Manchester and Manchester Children's University
Hospitals Trust
(Special interest: Respiratory Medicine)

Dr Tom Ledson MBChB MRCP
Registrar in Renal Medicine
Hope Hospital, Manchester

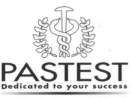

PASTEST
Dedicated to your success

© 2002 PASTEST Ltd
Egerton Court
Parkgate Estate
Knutsford
Cheshire
WA16 8DX

Telephone: 01565 752000

First published 2002

ISBN: 1 901198 58 8

A catalogue record for this book is available from the British Library.

The information contained within this book was obtained by the authors from reliable sources. However, while every effort has been made to ensure its accuracy, no responsibility for loss, damage or injury occasioned to any person acting or refraining from action as a result of information contained herein can be accepted by the publishers or authors.

PasTest Revision Books and Intensive Courses

PasTest has been established in the field of postgraduate medical education since 1972, providing revision books and intensive study courses for doctors preparing for their professional examinations. Books and courses are available for the following specialties:

MRCGP, MRCP Part 1 and 2, MRCPCH Part 1 and 2, MRCPsych, MRCS, MRCOG, DRCOG, DCH, FRCA, PLAB.

For further details contact:

PasTest, Freepost, Knutsford, Cheshire WA16 7BR
Tel: 01565 752000 Fax: 01565 650264
www.pastest.co.uk   enquiries@pastest.co.uk

Text prepared by Vision Typesetting, Manchester
Printed and bound in Great Britain by Page Bros (Norwich) Ltd

Contents

Introduction

This book is a compilation of clinical, diagnostic, investigative and prognostic features of the symptoms and diseases that cover the whole spectrum of general medicine.

It is aimed at the MRCP candidate and provides comprehensive lists in the subject areas that commonly appear in both part 1 and part 2 of the exam. It will be particularly useful for last-minute revision and will also be a useful resource for doctors on the ward when they come across a clinical problem for which there are a number of possible causes.

Even though the MRCP exams do change, lists will remain a vital resource in the candidates' preparation. Although there are several revision books for the MRCP, there have so far been very few that are made up simply of lists. This book aims to fill that gap.

Every effort has been made to make the lists as 'user friendly' as possible and they are arranged systematically, the subjects in alphabetical order, with a useful list of abbreviations and a comprehensive index.

Try to memorise as much of each list as possible. You can do this by covering up each heading and reciting the list that follows. Test your colleagues and ask them to test you. If you think that the lists are too long, then break them down into what you think is necessary for your particular needs. Writing your own list will help you to remember more easily.

Finally, we would like to acknowledge the contribution made by Dr Rachel Argyle to the cardiology chapter.

List of Abbreviations

AAFB	Acid-alcohol-fast bacilli
Ab	Antibody
ABPA	Allergic bronchopulmonary aspergillosis
ACE	Angiotensin-converting enzyme
ACTH	Adrenocorticotrophic hormone
AD	Autosomal dominant
ADH	Antidiuretic hormone
ADP	Adenosine diphosphate
AF	Atrial fibrillation
AFP	Alphafetoprotein
Ag	Antigen
ALL	Acute lymphoblastic leukaemia
ALP	Alkaline phosphatase
AML	Acute myeloid leukaemia
ANA	Antinuclear antibody
AP	Amyloid P component
APC	Antigen-presenting cell
APKD	Adult polycystic kidney disease
APML	Acute promyelocytic leukaemia
APPT	Activated partial thromboplastin time (with kaolin)
AR	Autosomal recessive
ARDS	Adult (or acute) respiratory distress syndrome
ARF	Acute renal failure
AS	Aortic stenosis
ASA	Amino salacyclic acid
ASD	Atrial septal defect
ASOT	Antistreptolysin-O titre
AST	Aspartate aminotransferase
ATN	Acute tubular necrosis
AV	Atrio-ventricular

AXR	Abdominal X-ray
BCC	Basal cell carcinoma
BCG	Bacillus Calmette–Guérin
BTS	British Thoracic Society
cANCA	Cytoplasmic-staining anti-neutrophil cytoplasmic antibody
CAPRIE	Clopidogrel v aspirin in patients at risk of ischaemic events
CAPTURE	Chimeric C7E3 anti-platelet therapy in unstable angina refractory to standard treatment trial
CCF	Congestive cardiac failure
CCK	Cholecystokinin
CEA	Carcinoembryonic antigen
CF	Cystic fibrosis
CFA	Cryptogenic fibrosing alveolitis
CFTR	Cystic fibrosis transmembrane regulator protein
CHB	Complete heart block
CJD	Creutzfeldt–Jakob disease
CLL	Chronic lymphocytic leukaemia
CML	Chronic myeloid leukaemia
CMML	Chronic myelomonocytic leukaemia
CMV	Cytomegalovirus
CNS	Central nervous system
COPD	Chronic obstructive pulmonary disease
CPAP	Continuous positive airway pressure
CPR	Cardiopulmonary resuscitation
CREST	Calcinosis, Raynaud's phenomenon, (o)esophageal dysfunction, sclerodactyly and telangiectasia
CRF	Chronic renal failure
CRH	Corticotrophin-releasing hormone
CRP	C-reactive protein
CSF	Cerebrospinal fluid
CT	Computerised tomography
CTD	Connective tissue disorder
CVA	Cerebrovascular accident
CXR	Chest X-ray
DAF	Decay activating factor
DEXA	Dual-energy X-ray absorptiometry
DIC	Disseminated intravascular coagulation
DKA	Diabetic ketoacidosis
DMSA	Dimercaptosuccinic acid
dsDNA	Double-stranded DNA
DTPA	Diethylenetriamine penta-acetic acid
DU	Duodenal ulcer
DVT	Deep vein thrombosis

EBV	Epstein–Barr virus
ECG	Electrocardiogram
EEG	Electroencephalography
EF	Ejection fraction
ELISA	Enzyme-linked immunosorbent assay
EMG	Electromyography
EPIC	Evaluation of 7E3 for the prevention of ischaemic complications trial
EPILOG	Evaluation in PTCA to improve longterm outcome with abciximab gpiib/iiia blockade
EPS	Electro physiological studies
ERCP	Endoscopic retrograde cholangiopancreatography
ESR	Erthrocyte sedimentation rate
ESRF	End-stage renal failure
FBC	Full blood counts
FEV_1	Forced expiratory volume (in one second)
FFP	Fresh frozen plasma
FSH	Follicle-stimulating hormone
FVC	Forced vital capacity
GBM	Glomerular basement membrane
G-CSF	Granulocyte colony-stimulating factor
GFR	Glomerular filtration rate
GH	Growth hormone
GHRH	Growth hormone-releasing hormone
GIP	Gastric inhibitory protein
GM-CSF	Granulocyte macrophage colony-stimulating factor
GMP	Guanosine monophosphate
GN	Glomerulonephritis
GORD	Gastro-oesophageal reflux disease
GTN	Glyceryl trinitrate
GU	Gastric ulcer
GVHD	Graft-versus-host disease
HBV	Hepatitis B virus
HCC	Hepatocellular carcinoma
HCG	Human chorionic gonadotrophin
HCM	Hypertrophic cardiomyopathy
HCV	Hepatitis C virus
HHV	Human herpes virus
HIV	Human immunodeficiency virus
HLA	Human leucocyte antigen
HCM	Hypertrophic obstructive cardiomyopathy
HONK	Hyperosmolar non-ketotic state
HPV	Human papilloma virus

HRT	Hormone replacement therapy
HSP	Henoch–Schönlein purpura
HSV	Herpes simplex virus
HTLV	Human T-cell lymphotropic virus
HUS	Haemolytic uraemic syndrome
IBS	Irritable bowel syndrome
ICAM	Intercellular adhesion molecule
ICP	Intracranial pressure
IDA	Iron deficiency anaemia
IDL	Intermediate density lipoprotein
IFN	Interferon
Ig	Immunoglobulin
IGF	Insulin-like growth factor
IHD	Ischaemic heart disease
IL	Interleukin
INR	International normalised ratio
ITP	Idiopathic thrombocytopenia
IUGR	Intrauterine growth retardation
JVP	Jugular venous pulse
LAD	Left axis deviation
LBBB	Left bundle branch block
LDL	Low density lipoprotein
LFT	Liver function test
LGL	Lown–Ganong–Levine syndrome
LH	Luteinising hormone
LICS	Left intercostal space
LPS	Lipopolysaccharide
LSE	Left sternal edge
LV	Left ventricle
LVH	Left ventricular hypertrophy
MAC	Membrane attack complex
MAG3	Mercaptoacetyltriglycine (in 99mTc-MAG3)
MALT	Mucosa-associated lymphoid tissue
MAOI	Monoamine oxidase inhibitor
MCGN	Mesangiocapillary glomerulonephritis
MCH	Mean corpuscular haemoglobin
MCP	Metacarpophalangeal (joints)
MCTD	Mixed connective tissue disease
MCV	Mean corpuscular volume (of red cells)
MEN	Multiple endocrine neoplasia
MG	Myasthenia gravis
MGUS	Monoclonal gammopathy of unknown significance
MI	Myocardial infarction

MIBG	Metaiodobenzylguanidiene
MIP	Macrophage inhibitory protein
MMR	Measles, mumps and rubella
MMSE	Mini mental state examination
MND	Motor neurone disease
MR	Mitral regurgitation
MPTP	1-methyl-4-phenyl-1,2,3,6-tetrahydropyridine
MRCP	Magnetic resonance cholangiopancreatography
MRI	Magnetic resonance imaging
MRSA	Methicillin-resistant *Staphylococcus aureus*
MTP	Metatarsophalangeal (joints)
MV	Mitral valve
MVP	Mitral valve prolapse
NADPH	(reduced form of) Nicotinamide-adenine dinucleotide phosphate
NHL	Non-Hodgkin's lymphoma
NSAID	Non-steroidal anti-inflammatory drugs
OA	Osteoarthritis
OCP	Oral contraceptive pill
PA	Pernicious anaemia
PABA	Para-aminobenzoic acid
PAN	Polyarteritis nodosa
pANCA	Perinuclear-staining anti-neutrophil cytoplasmic antibody
PBC	Primary biliary cirrhosis
PCOS	Polycystic ovarian syndrome
PCP	*Pneumocystis carinii* pneumonia
PDA	Patent ductus arteriosus
PE	Pulmonary embolus
PEA	Pulseless electrical activity
PEEP	Positive end-expiratory pressure
PEFR	Peak expiratory flow rate
PIP	Proximal interphalangeal (joints)
PMF	Progressive massive fibrosis
PML	Progressive multifocal leucoencephalopathy
PMR	Polymyalgia rheumatica
PPI	Proton pump inhibitor
PPP	Pancreatic polypeptide
PS	Pulmonary stenosis
PSC	Primary sclerosing cholangitis
PT	Prothrombin time
PTH	Parathyroid hormone
PTHrP	Parathyroid hormone-related protein
PVD	Peripheral vascular disease

RA	Rheumatoid arthritis
RAA	Renin-angiotensin-aldosterone (axis or system)
RAD	Right axis deviation
RBBB	Right bundle branch block
RICS	Right intercostal space
RNP	Ribonucleoprotein
RSV	Respiratory syncytial virus
RTA	Renal tubular acidosis
SBE	Subacute bacterial endocarditis
Se HCAT	23-selena H,25-homotaurocholate
sens.	Sensitivity
SI	Sacroiliac
SIADH	Syndrome of inappropriate ADH secretion
SLE	Systemic lupus erythematosis
SMA	Smooth muscle antibody
spec.	Specificity
SSRI	Selective serotonin-reuptake inhibitors
STD	Sexually transmitted disease
SVC	Superior vena cava
TCA	Tricyclic antidepressant
TGF	Transforming growth factor
TIBC	Total iron-binding capacity
TIPS	Transjugular intrahepatic portocaval shunt
TLC	Total lung capacity
TMJ	Temporomandibular joint
TNF	Tumour necrosis factor
TR	Tricuspid regurgitation
TRH	Thyrotrophin-releasing hormone
TT	Thrombin time
TTP	Thrombotic thrombocytopenic purpura
TSH	Thyroid-stimulating hormone
TV	Tidal volume
USS	Ultrasound scan
VC	Vital capacity
VDRL	Venereal Disease Research Laboratories (test, for syphilis)
VIP	Vasoactive intestinal polypeptide
VLDL	Very low density lipoprotein
VSD	Ventricular septal defect
VT	Ventricular tachycardia
VZV	Varicella zoster virus
WCC	White cell count
WPW	Wolff–Parkinson–White syndrome
ZN	Ziehl–Neelsen (stain)

Jo-1, La, Ro and Sm are fractions of nuclear material.

AIDS HIV Medicine

MODES OF TRANSMISSION

1 Sexual intercourse (vaginal/anal) – heterosexual, male homosexual. Risk with oral sex is minimal
2 IV drug abuse using shared needles plus equipment
3 Blood transfusion and other blood products
4 Maternal–fetal transmisson – delivery by caesarean section reduces risk; avoid breastfeeding.

THE VIRUS

1 The human immunodeficiency virus (HIV) is a human retrovirus, a member of the lentivirus family
2 An RNA virus, it contains enzyme reverse transcriptase
3 There are two known types: HIV-1, which is prevalent worldwide, and HIV-2, common in West Africa
4 HIV has an affinity for the following CD4 cells:
   (a) helper T lymphocytes
   (b) B lymphocytes
   (c) macrophages
   (d) CNS cells
5 Causes progressive immune dysfunction, characterised by CD4-cell depletion.

SEROCONVERSION

After innoculation seroconversion can take up to six months (the 'window period'), when HIV antibody may not be detectable.

Symptoms of seroconversion illness

1 Fever
2 Malaise
3 Diarrhoea
4 Meningoencephalitis
5 Rash
6 Sore throat
7 Lymphadenopathy
8 Arthralgia.

CENTERS FOR DISEASE CONTROL (CDC) CLASSIFICATION OF AIDS

Stage 1 – primary seroconversion illness
Stage 2 – asymptomatic
Stage 3 – persistent generalised lymphadenopathy
Stage 4a – AIDS-related complex (fever, weight loss, malaise, diarrhoea but no features of AIDS indicator illnesses)
Stages 4b–d AIDS – patients develop opportunistic infections or tumours (AIDS indicator illnesses).

BASELINE INVESTIGATIONS FOR NEW DIAGNOSIS OF HIV INFECTION

1 *Microbiology:*
   (a) syphilis serology
   (b) toxoplasmosis serology
   (c) cryptococcal antigen
   (d) screen for other STDs
2 *Virology:*
   (a) HIV antibody (confirmatory test)
   (b) p24 antigen/antibody and viral lode
   (c) hepatitis serology (B and C)
   (d) cytomegalovirus (CMV) antibody
3 *Haematology:*
   (a) FBC (differential and film)

(b) ESR
4 *Biochemistry:* liver and renal function tests
5 *Immunology:*
   (a) lymphocyte subsets (CD4 count)
   (b) neopterin
   (c) β_2-microglobulin
6 CXR
7 Lung function tests
8 Cervical cytology.

INDICATOR DISEASES FOR AIDS

1 Recurrent bacterial chest infections (in a 12-month period)
2 Candidiasis (trachea, bronchi, lungs, oesphagus)
3 Invasive carcinoma of the cervix
4 Coccidioidomycosis, disseminated or extrapulmonary
5 *Cryptococcus* infection, extrapulmonary
6 Cryptosporidiosis with diarrhoea for more than one month
7 Cytomegalovirus disease (not in liver, spleen or nodes)
8 Encephalopathy (primary progressive dementia) due to HIV
9 Herpes simplex ulcers for more than one month (genital, oral, occasionally disseminated) or bronchitis, pneumonitis, or oesophagitis
10 Histoplasmosis, disseminated or extrapulmonary
11 Isosporiosis with diarrhoea for more than one month
12 Kaposi's sarcoma
13 Lymphoid interstitial pneumonitis and/or pulmonary lymphoid hyperplasia (in children under 13 years)
14 Mycobacteriosis, pulmonary TB
15 *Pneumocystis carinii* pneumonia (PCP)
16 Progressive multifocal leucoencephalopathy
17 Recurrent *Salmonella* (non-typhoid) septicaemia
18 Toxoplasma infection (cerebral) after one month of age
19 Wasting syndrome (over 10% loss with no other cause identified).

DRUG THERAPIES IN HIV/AIDS

The aims of treatment are:

1 Complete suppression of viral replication
2 A synergistic effect with combination therapy
3 Reduction of the risk of emergence of viral resistance.

Nucleoside reverse transcriptase inhibitors (NRTIs)

1 Zidovudine (AZT)
2 Lamivudine (3TC)
3 Didanosine (DDI)
4 Stavudine.

Non-nucleoside reverse transcriptase inhibitors (NNRTIs)

1 Nevirapine
2 Efavirenz.

Protease inhibitors (PIs)

1 Indinavir
2 Ritonavir
3 Saquinavir
4 Nelfinavir.

Treatment strategies

1 The decision to start treatment depends on:
   (a) CD4 count
   (b) plasma viral load
   (c) clinical symptoms
2 Three drugs are used, including two NRTIs and *either* one PI *or* one NNRTI
3 Beneficial effects must be balanced against drug toxicity (including irreversible damage to the immune system) and the development of viral drug resistance
4 This is an area of rapid change – i.e. consult an expert.

RESPIRATORY DISEASE IN HIV/AIDS

Pneumocystis carinii pneumonia

1 A common presentation

2 Abnormal CXR in 90%
3 Hypoxic
4 Dry cough, fever, malaise
5 Treatment is with high-dose co-trimoxazole.

Pulmonary TB

1 Very common presenting illness in sub-Saharan Africa
2 Extrapulmonary disease is more common in these
   immunocompromised patients
3 Does not tend to show classic CXR changes
4 Multi-drug resistance is likely in HIV/AIDS patients
5 Atypical mycobacterium infections may occur, e.g. *M. avium
   intracellulare*
6 Development is unrelated to the CD4 count.

Viral infections

1 CMV (retinitis, colitis, oesophagitis, encephalitis, pneumonitis)
2 HSV
3 Epstein–Barr virus (EBV)
4 Adenovirus
5 Influenza virus.

Bacterial infections

1 *Streptococcus pneumoniae*
2 *Staphylococcus aureus*
3 *Mycobacterium tuberculosis* and *M. avium intracellulare*.

Fungal infections

1 *Candida*
2 Histoplasmosis
3 *Cryptococcus*
4 *Nocardia*.

Tumours

1 Kaposi's sarcoma
2 Non-Hodgkin's lymphoma.

GASTROINTESTINAL DISEASE IN HIV/AIDS
(see also pages 170–171)

Oropharyngeal/Oesophageal disease

99% of patients will develop oral/oesophageal problems:
1 Candidiasis
2 Oral hairy leukoplakia
3 Aphthous ulcer
4 Periodontal disease
5 HSV infection
6 Lymphoma
7 Kaposi's sarcoma
8 CMV infection.

Diarrhoeal disease

May be caused by:
1 Bacteria:
    (a) *Salmonella*
    (b) *Campylobacter*
    (c) *Shigella*
2 Protozoa – *Giardia lamblia*, amoeba
3 Virus – CMV
4 Opportunistic organisms:
    (a) bacteria – atypical mycobacteria
    (b) protozoa – *Isospora belli, Cryptosporidium, Microsporidium*.

Gastrointestinal neoplasms

1 Kaposi's sarcoma
2 Intraabdominal lymphoma.

Bilary and pancreatic disease

1 Cholangiopathy – due to drugs, *Cryptosporidium,* CMV or *Microsporidium*
2 Pancreatitis – as above.

Anorectal conditions

Symptoms include:

1 Tenesmus
2 Pruritus ani
3 Rectal bleeding
4 Diarrhoea.

Causative agents:

1 HSV
2 Wart virus
3 *Treponema pallidum*
4 *Neisseria gonorrhoeae*
5 *Chlamydia*.

NEUROLOGIAL DISEASE IN HIV/AIDS

1 Can be the first presentation of the disease in up to 10% of patients
2 May present with lymphocytic meningitis
3 Presents with focal signs or generalised features but is often asymptomatic.

Direct neurotropic effects

1 AIDS-dementia complex – now less common with antiretroviral therapy
2 Vacuolar myelopathy
3 Neuropathy.

Neurological infections

Focal disease

1 *Mycobacterium tuberculosis* (meningitis, abscess)
2 *Toxoplasma gondii.*

Generalised disease

1 *Cryptococcus neoformans* (meningitis)
2 CMV (retinitis, peripheral neuropathy)
3 Polyonav virus – JC virus (progressive multifocal leucoencephalopathy).

Neurosyphilis

Can cause aggressive and atypical neurosyphilis, with:
1 Myelopathy
2 Retinitis
3 Meningitis
4 Meningovascular complications.

OPHTHALMIC COMPLICATIONS OF HIV/AIDS

1 Molluscum contagiosum of the lids
2 Episcleritis and keratitis
3 Uveitis
4 Kaposi's sarcoma (lids or conjunctiva)
5 Retinal changes – haemorrhages, cotton wool spots, oedema, vascular sheathing
6 Choroidal granulomas
7 CMV retinitis
8 Toxoplasmosis
9 *Candida* endophthalmitis
10 Neuro-ophthalmic manifestations.

DERMATOLOGICAL COMPLICATIONS OF HIV/AIDS

Affect up to 75% of all patients with HIV. During seroconversion patients may develop a marked seborrhoeic dermatitis. As the disease progresses atypical infections and tumours are seen:
1 *General dermatoses:*
  (a) psoriasis
  (b) eczema
  (c) seborrhoeic dermatitis
  (d) folliculitis
2 *Fungal/yeast infections:*
  (a) *Pityrosporum ovale*
  (b) Candidiasis*
  (c) *Cryptococcus neoformans*
  (d) *Histoplasma capsulatum*
3 Viral infections:

(a) HSV/VZV infections
(b) EBV
(c) human papilloma virus*
(d) CMV
(e) molluscum contagiosum*
4 *Bacterial infections:*
(a) TB
(b) syphilis
(c) *Staphylococcus aureus*
(d) bacillary angiomatosis
5 *Malignancy:*
(a) Kaposi's sarcoma
(b) lymphomas
(c) cervical intraepithelial neoplasia
(d) oral squamous carcinoma.

*Most common infections.

Cardiology

PULSES

Collapsing pulse (waterhammer or Corrigan's pulse)

Large amplitude; rapid rise and fall.
1 Aortic regurgitation
2 Severe anaemia
3 Patent ductus arteriosus
4 AV shunt
5 Hyperthyroidism
6 Heart block.

Small-volume pulse (pulsus parvus)

Thready.
1 Cardiac failure
2 Hypovolaemia (shock)
3 Vasoconstriction
4 Reduced cardiac output due to obstruction:
   (a) any valve stenosis
   (b) pulmonary hypertension.

Pulsus paradoxus

Exaggeration of the normal fall in pulse volume with respiration.
1 Cardiac tamponade
2 Constrictive pericarditis
3 Obstructive airways disease (asthma or chronic bronchitis)
4 Massive pulmonary embolus.

Pulsus bisferiens (double peak)

First component is from a large systolic blood ejection; second component is due to arterial elastic recoil.

1 Combined aortic stenosis and regurgitation
2 Hypertrophic cardiomyopathy (rarely).

Pulsus alternans

Alternating large- and small-volume beats (uncommon). Occurs in left ventricular failure.

Slow-rising pulse

Delayed percussion wave. Occurs in aortic stenosis.

Absent radial pulse

1 Aortic dissection with subclavian involvement
2 Congenital
3 Iatrogenic (surgery or catheterisation)
4 Arterial embolism
5 Takayasu's arteritis
6 Trauma.

JVP

Large a waves

1 Pulmonary hypertension
2 Pulmonary stenosis
3 Tricuspid stenosis.

Absent a waves

1 AF

Large v waves

1 Tricuspid regurgitation

Cannon waves

1 Complete heart block
2 Extrasystoles
3 Nodal rhythm.

HEART SOUNDS

First heart sound

Closure of mitral and tricuspid valves.

Loud

1 Mobile mitral stenosis
2 Hyperdynamic states
3 Tachycardia
4 Left to right shunts
5 Short PR interval (e.g. WPW, LGL).

Soft

1 Immobile mitral stenosis
2 MR
3 Impaired LV function
4 Prolonged PR interval.

Variable

Any cause of AV dissociation.
1 CHB
2 VT
3 AF.

Split

1 RBBB
2 LBBB
3 VT
4 Inspiration
5 ASD
6 Tricuspid stenosis.

Second heart sound

Closure of aortic and then pulmonary valves.

Loud

1 Systemic hypertension (loud A2)
2 Pulmonary hypertension (loud P2)
3 Tachycardia
4 ASD (loud P2).

Soft

1 Severe AS
2 Aortic root dilatation.

Wide splitting

Late P2

1 Inspiration (physiological)
2 RBBB
3 Prolonged RV systole (e.g. PE, pulmonary stenosis)
4 ASD (fixed splitting, doesn't vary with respiration).

Early A2

Shortened LV systole (e.g. MR, VSD).

Reversed splitting

Late A2

1 Expiration
2 LBBB
3 Prolonged LV systole (e.g. HCM, IHD, PDA, AS).

Early P2

WPW (type B).

Single S2

1 Severe AS/PS
2 Large VSD
3 Hypertension
4 Tetralogy of Fallot

5 Eisenmenger's syndrome
6 Pulmonary atresia
7 Advanced age.

Third heart sound

Best heard at left sternal edge or apex.
1 *Physiological*, due to passive ventricular filling on opening of the AV valves:
   (a) young people (<40 years)
   (b) pregnancy
   (c) hyperdynamic states (e.g. thyrotoxicosis)
2 *Pathological*, due to rapid ventricular filling:
   (a) LVF
   (b) cardiomyopathy
   (c) MR
   (d) VSD
   (e) constrictive pericarditis.

Fourth heart sound

Always pathological. Due to the increased atrial contraction required to fill a stiff left ventricle. Does not occur in atrial fibrillation.
1 LVH
2 Following MI
3 Amyloid heart disease
4 HCM.

MURMURS

Systolic murmurs

Mid-systolic murmurs

1 Innocent flow murmur:
   (a) soft, short murmur
   (b) left sternal edge or pulmonary area
   (c) no other abnormalities on examination, ECG or CXR

2 Aortic stenosis or sclerosis:
   (a) aortic area (2nd RICS), radiating to neck, and/or left sternal
       edge/apex
   (b) often associated with a thrill
3 Pulmonary stenosis:
   (a) 2nd LICS
   (b) increased on inspiration
   (c) quiet and delayed P2
   (d) may have a click
4 Coarctation of the aorta:
   (a) loud, coarse murmur
   (b) maximal over apex of left lung (anterior and posterior)
5 Hypertrophic cardiomyopathy: increased by Valsalva manoeuvre
6 Atrial septal defect (high pulmonary flow):
   (a) fixed split S2
   (b) possible associated diastolic murmur if ASD is large
7 Tetralogy of Fallot.

Pan-systolic murmurs

1 Mitral regurgitation: apex, radiating to axilla
2 Tricuspid regurgitation:
   (a) left sternal edge
   (b) low-pitched
3 Ventricular septal defect:
   (a) left sternal edge
   (b) harsh.

Late systolic murmurs

1 Mitral valve prolapse (apex)
2 Hypertrophic cardiomyopathy.

Diastolic murmurs

Early diastolic murmurs

1 Aortic regurgitation:
   (a) often associated with mitral stenosis
   (b) blowing quality
   (c) maximal 3rd LICS in expiration

(d) radiates to right carotid or apex
2 Pulmonary regurgitation:
    (a) very rare
    (b) blowing quality
    (c) maximal 2nd/3rd LICS
3 Graham Steell murmur: pulmonary regurgitation secondary to pulmonary hypertension and mitral stenosis.

Mid-diastolic murmurs

1 Mitral stenosis:
    (a) mid-late diastole
    (b) rumbling quality
    (c) apex
2 Austin Flint murmur:
    (a) aortic regurgitant jet, impairing diastolic flow through the mitral valve
    (b) left sternal edge
3 Carey Coombs murmur: due to rheumatic fever
4 High AV flow states: ASD, VSD, PDA, anaemia, MR, TR
5 Atrial tumours: especially if disturbing flow across the aortic valve
6 Tricuspid stenosis.

Continuous murmurs

Maximal in systole but persistent into diastole.
1 Patent ductus arteriosus:
    (a) 2nd LICS, mid-clavicular line
    (b) machinery-like quality
    (c) also audible posteriorly
2 Venous hum: positional
3 AV shunts/fistulae (in lungs or coronary arteries)
4 Ruptured sinus of Valsalva: high pitched due to high pressure
5 ASD
6 Mixed aortic valve disease.

ARRHYTHMIAS

Tachyarrhythmias

Sinus tachycardia

Rate > 100 b.p.m.
1 Anxiety
2 Fever
3 Pregnancy
4 Shock
5 Anaemia
6 CCF
7 Thyrotoxicosis
8 Phaeochromocytoma
9 Drugs, e.g. beta-agonists, vasodilators, atropine
10 Constrictive pericarditis (rarely).

Paroxysmal atrial tachycardia

Rate 120–200 b.p.m.
1 Idiopathic
2 Thyrotoxicosis
3 Digoxin and other drugs (e.g. tobacco, caffeine).

Atrial flutter or fibrillation (AF)

Ventricular rate > 100 b.p.m. (irregular if fibrillation).
1 Idiopathic ('lone AF')
2 MI
3 IHD
4 Valvular heart disease (especially mitral stenosis)
5 Hypertension
6 Hyperthyroidism
7 Alcohol (and other drugs)
8 Cardiomyopathy (especially dilated)
9 Congenital heart disease
10 PE
11 Pericarditis (constrictive, or infiltrating neoplasm)
12 Pneumonia
13 Bronchial carcinoma (rarely)
14 ASD.

Junctional tachycardia (SVT)

Rate 140–220 b.p.m.
1 AV nodal re-entry tachycardia (usually in structurally normal hearts)
2 AV re-entry tachycardia (e.g. Wolff–Parkinson–White syndrome).

Ventricular tachycardia (VT)

Rate 140–220 b.p.m.
1 Myocardial infarction or chronic IHD
2 Myocarditis
3 Cardiomyopathy
4 Hyper- or hypokalaemia
5 Left ventricular aneurysm
6 Prolonged QT interval (see later) – predisposes to polymorphic VT ('torsades de pointes')
7 Congenital abnormalities of the RV outflow tract – VT with LBBB and RAD
8 Mitral valve prolapse.

Features suggesting VT rather than SVT in broad-complex tachycardia:
1 History of IHD
2 AV dissociation
3 Capture beats
4 Fusion beats
5 QRS > 0.14 s
6 Extreme LAD
7 Concordance of QRS complexes across chest leads
8 No response to adenosine or carotid sinus massage
9 QRS morphology different from that found in sinus rhythm.

Bradyarrhythmias

Sinus bradycardia

Rate 40–50 b.p.m.
1 Athleticism
2 Myocardial infarction
3 Hypothyroidism
4 Hypothermia
5 Sinus node disease

6 Cholestatic jaundice
7 Raised ICP
8 Increased vagal tone e.g. vomiting
9 Drugs (e.g. beta-blockers, digoxin, verapamil).

Complete heart block (third-degree AV block)

1 25–50 b.p.m. (ventricular escape rhythm)
2 Rate does not vary with exercise (except congenital form)
3 Narrow (more stable) or wide QRS complexes
4 Associated with large-volume pulse and systolic flow murmurs.

CHB may be:
1 *Congenital*, or
2 *Acquired:*
   (a) idiopathic fibrosis
   (b) MI/IHD
   (c) acute inflammation (e.g. endocarditis)
   (d) chronic inflammation (e.g. sarcoid)
   (e) drugs (e.g. rate-limiting agents)
   (f) trauma.

Indications for permanent pacemakers

1 Complete heart block
2 Mobitz 2 heart block
3 Sinus node dysfunction
4 Symptomatic sinus bradycardia
5 Bifasicular and trifasicular block accompanied by syncope
6 Hypertrophic cardiomyopathy
7 Post AV nodal ablation for arrythmias.

Indications for AICDs (NICE guidelines)

Primary prevention

1 Post MI with
   (a) non-sustained VT on 24 hour tape
   (b) inducible VT on EPS studies
   (c) left ventricular dysfunction (EF < 35%)
2 Familial cardiac condition
   (a) long QT interval

(b) hypertrophic cardiomyopathy
(c) Brugada syndrome (RBBB and downsloping ST elevation in V1)
(d) arrythmogenic right ventricular dysplasia
(e) following repair of Fallot's tetralogy.

Secondary prevention

1 Cardiac arrest from VT or VF
2 Spontaneous VT causing significant haemodynamic compromise
3 Sustained VT with EF <35%.

Causes of syncope

Cardiac

1 Sinus node disease
2 Atrioventricular disease
3 Tachycardia
4 Bradycardia
5 Myocardial ischaemia
6 Aortic stenosis
7 Hypertrophic cardiomyopathy
8 Pulmonary hypertension
9 Pulmonary embolus
10 Atrial myxoma
11 Aortic dissection.

Neurogenic

1 Epilepsy
2 Vertibrobasilar ischaemia
3 Carotid artery stenosis (bilateral).

Others

1 Hypoglycaemia
2 Vasovagal syncope
3 Vasodilator drugs
4 Postural hypotension
   (a) elderly
   (b) Parkinson's disease
5 Autonomic neuropathy

6 Micturition syncope
7 Cough syncope
8 Carotid sinus hypersensitivity.

ECG ABNORMALITIES

Left bundle branch block (LBBB)

Almost always pathological.
1 Ischaemic heart disease
2 LVH
3 Hypertension
4 Aortic valve disease
5 Cardiomyopathy
6 Myocarditis
7 Post-valve replacement
8 RV pacemaker.

Right bundle branch block (RBBB)

May be a normal variant.
1 Physiological
2 RVH/RV strain (e.g. pulmonary embolus)
3 IHD
4 Congenital heart disease (e.g. ASD)
5 Myocarditis.

Broad-complex tachycardia

Rate > 140 b.p.m.; QRS > 0.12 s. (See section on
arrhythmias for distinguishing features.)
1 Ventricular tachycardia
2 SVT with bundle branch block.

Left axis deviation (LAD)

Deviation of − 30 to − 90 degrees; QRS negative in lead II.
1 LBBB
2 LVH
3 Left anterior hemiblock

4 Inferior MI
5 ASD (ostium primum type)
6 Cardiomyopathy
7 Artificial pacemaker
8 Tricuspid atresia.

Right axis deviation (RAD)

Deviation of +90 to +180 degrees; QRS negative in lead I.
1 Physiological in infants
2 RBBB
3 Right ventricular hypertrophy:
   (a) cor pulmonale
   (b) pulmonary embolism
   (c) mitral valve disease
   (d) pulmonary hypertension
   (e) pulmonary stenosis
   (f) tetralogy of Fallot
4 Anterolateral MI
5 Ostium secundum ASD
6 Left posterior hemiblock.

Short PR interval

Rarely < 0.12 s.
1 Wolff–Parkinson–White syndrome
2 Lown–Ganong–Levine syndrome
3 Concealed accessory pathway
4 P wave followed by ventricular ectopic
5 AV junctional rhythm (P wave usually negative)
6 Low atrial rhythm
7 Coronary sinus escape rhythm.

Wolff–Parkinson–White syndrome

1 Accessory pathway between atria and ventricles
2 Delta wave on ECG
3 Short PR interval
4 Type A – left side +ve R wave in V1
5 Type B – right side –ve R wave in V1
6 Arrythmias caused:

(a) AF
(b) SVT
(c) Sinus node dysfunction
(d) VF.

Prolonged QT interval

QT > 0.54 ms (normally 0.38–0.46 ms); associated with syncope and sudden death (from VT, especially polymorphic VT); 90% inherited.

1 Familial:
   (a) Romano–Ward syndrome (autosomal dominant)
   (b) Jervell and Lange–Nielsen syndrome (autosomal recessive)
2 IHD
3 Metabolic:
   (a) hypocalcaemia
   (b) hypokalaemia
   (c) hypomagnesaemia
   (d) hypothermia
   (e) hypothyroidism
4 Drugs, including:
   (a) erythromycin
   (b) amiodarone
   (c) terfenadine (and other antihistamines)
   (d) tricyclics
   (e) phenothiazines
   (f) quinine/quinidine
   (g) sotalol
5 Mitral valve prolapse
6 Rheumatic fever.

Dominant 'R' in V1

1 Right bundle branch block
2 Right ventricular hypertrophy
3 Posterior MI
4 Dextrocardia
5 Wolff–Parkinson–White type A – accessory pathway on left and posterior
6 HCM – septal mass is thicker than the posterior wall
7 Duchenne muscular dystrophy.

ST depression

1 Myocardial ischaemia (including posterior MI)
2 Digoxin therapy
3 Hypertension
4 LVH with strain
5 Hypokalaemia.

ST elevation

1 Myocardial infarction
2 Pericarditis
3 Left ventricular aneurysm
4 Coronary artery spasm (variant or Prinzmetal's angina)
5 Hyperkalaemia
6 Subarachnoid haemorrhage (rarely).

T-wave inversion

1 Ischaemia
2 Digoxin therapy
3 LVH
4 Cardiomyopathy
5 PE
6 Hypokalaemia (occasionally).

Pulseless electrical activity (PEA)

Previously known as 'electromechanical dissociation' or EMD, this is a cardiac arrest situation. A cardiac rhythm compatible with an output but without any palpable pulse.

1 Hypo- or hyperkalaemia (or other electrolyte disturbances)
2 Hypothermia
3 Hypovolaemia
4 Hypoxia
5 Cardiac tamponade
6 Tension pneumothorax
7 Pulmonary embolus
8 Drug overdose/toxins
9 Aortic dissection
10 Myocardial infarction.

CARDIOMYOPATHIES

Dilated cardiomyopathy

Global ventricular dilatation and dysfunction; more common in males and in Afro-Caribbeans.

1 Hereditary (30%)
   (a) X-linked
   (b) autosomal dominant
2 Alcohol
3 Ischaemia
4 Viruses:
   (a) Coxsackie
   (b) HIV
5 Pregnancy
6 Drugs – anthracyclines
7 Hypertension (untreated)
8 Autoimmune disease:
   (a) hyper- and hypothyroidism
   (b) diabetes
9 Nutritional deficiencies (e.g. thiamine deficiency)
10 Muscular dystrophies
11 Friedreich's ataxia.

Restrictive cardiomyopathy

Stiff, rigid ventricles lead to impaired diastolic filling.

1 Idiopathic
2 Amyloidosis
3 Endomyocardial fibrosis
4 Loeffler's syndrome (and other eosinophilias)
5 Carcinoid syndrome
6 Infiltrations
   (a) sarcoidosis
   (b) haemachromatosis
   (c) Gaucher's disease
   (d) Fabry's disease
7 Connective tissue disorders (e.g. SLE, PAN, systemic sclerosis)
8 Malignancy
9 Radiotherapy
10 Drugs.

Hypertrophic cardiomyopathy (HCM)

Autosomal dominant
Asymmetric hypertrophy of left or right ventricle, or both.
1 Clinical features
   (a) breathlessness
   (b) chest pains
   (c) collapse/syncope
   (d) palpitations (AF, SVT, VT)
   (e) sudden death
2 Signs
   (a) jerky pulse
   (b) forceful apex
   (c) prominent a wave in JVP
   (d) 4th heart sound (not AF)
   (e) ejection systolic murmur (increased by squatting)
3 Treatment
   (a) amiodarone
   (b) digoxin (AF)
   (c) anticoagulation (AF)
   (d) beta blockers
   (e) verapamil
   (f) permanent pacemakers
   (g) implantable defibrillators.

PERICARDIAL DISEASES

Acute pericarditis

1 Post MI: Dressler's syndrome (rare), characterised by fever,
   pleurisy, pericarditis and the formation of antibodies to heart muscle –
   occurs two weeks to two months post MI or cardiac surgery
2 Infective:
   (a) viral (most common), e.g. Coxsackie B virus
   (b) bacterial
   (c) Tuberculosis
3 Rheumatic fever
4 Severe uraemia
5 Malignancy (e.g. lymphoma, breast or bronchial carcinoma)

6 Trauma

7 Connective tissue disorders (e.g. SLE)

8 Hypothyroidism.

Constrictive pericarditis

1 Postinfective (bacterial or viral) pericarditis

2 Recurrent pericarditis

3 Connective tissue disorders (e.g. rheumatoid arthritis)

4 Trauma (haemopericardium)

5 Cardiac surgery

6 TB

7 Radiotherapy to the mediastinum

8 Drugs

9 Malignancy

10 Severe uraemic pericarditis.

Pericardial effusion and cardiac tamponade

1 Any cause of constrictive pericarditis

2 Ventricular rupture (due to IHD)

3 Iatrogenic (cardiac pacing/catheterisation)

4 Aortic dissection

5 Anticoagulation with acute pericarditis.

DRUGS AND THE HEART

(see also Clinical Pharmacology)

Side-effects of amiodarone

These are some of the most common and most clinically significant:

1 Thyroid problems (hyper- or hypothyroidism)

2 Photosensitivity

3 Liver toxicity (hepatitic picture)

4 Peripheral neuropathy

5 Pulmonary fibrosis

6 Corneal microdeposits (cause glaring of headlights at night; reversible when drug is stopped)

7 Metallic taste

8 Skin discoloration
9 Ataxia
10 Arrhythmias (especially torsades).

Digoxin toxicity

1 Arrhythmias (especially AV block)
2 Nausea and vomiting
3 Diarrhoea
4 Headaches
5 Anorexia
6 Xanthopsia (yellow vision)
7 Seizures
8 Neuralgia
9 Impotence
10 Skin reactions.

Antiarrythmic drugs

Class 1

Inhibit inward sodium channels.
1 *1a* (quinidine, disopyramide and procainamide)
   (a) lengthen action potential
   (b) prolong QT interval
   (c) used in treatment of VT and to cardiovert AF
2 *1b* (lignocaine)
   (a) shortens cardiac action potential
   (b) treatment of VT and prophylaxis of VT/VF
3 *1c* (Flecainide)
   (a) Prolongs QT
   (b) no change in cardiac action potential
   (c) negatively ionotropic
   (d) used in AF cardioversion, AF prophylaxis, VT prophylaxis and WPW.

Class 2

Beta blockers
1 Negatively ionotropic
2 Antagonise catacholamines
3 Used in AF rate controls, AF prophylaxis and SVT prophylaxis.

Class 3

Sotalol
1 Prolongs QT
2 Beta blocker activity
3 Used in AF termination, AF and VT prophylaxis and WPW prophylaxis.
Amiodarone
1 Prolongs QT
2 Used in AF termination, AF and VT prophylaxis and WPW prophylaxis
3 Side effects – see above.

Class 4

Verapamil
1 reduces inward current of calcium in SA or AV nodes
2 Negatively ionotropic
3 Used in SVT termination, SVT prophylaxis and AF rate control.

Others

Adenosine
1 Causes transient AV block
2 Will terminate arrythmias involving the AV node (SVT)
3 Very short half-life
4 Half life-prolonged by dipyridamole leading to asystole
5 Causes chest tightness and bronchospasm.

ISCHAEMIC HEART DISEASE (IHD)

Risk factors

1 Hypertension
2 Diabetes
3 Smoking
4 Hypercholesterolaemia ($\uparrow$ LDL, $\uparrow$ TG, $\downarrow$ HDL)
5 Family history of premature heart disease
6 Chronic renal failure
7 Obesity
8 Male gender
9 Increasing age

10 Alcohol excess
11 Sedentary lifestyle
12 Drugs (contraceptive pill)
13 Ethnicity (Afro-Caribbean – low, Indo-Asians – high)
14 Type A personality
15 ↑Lipoprotein a
16 ↑Homocysteine levels
17 ↑Fibrinogen.

Complications of MI

1 Arrhythmias – VT/VF, CHB or other AV block
2 Heart failure/cardiogenic shock
3 Hypertension
4 Thromboembolic disease
5 Pericarditis or Dressler's syndrome
6 VSD
7 Mitral regurgitation
8 Papillary muscle rupture
9 Cardiac rupture
10 LV aneurysm.

Contraindications to thrombolysis

These are a guide only; some are absolute and some only relative
contraindications, depending on the clinical circumstances:
1 Internal bleeding
2 Recent surgery (including liver or kidney biopsy) or trauma (within
   the last two weeks)
3 Suspected aortic dissection or aneurysm
4 Recent head injury (within two weeks)
5 Intracranial neoplasm
6 Previous proven haemorrhagic CVA
7 BP > 200/120
8 Active diabetic proliferative retinopathy
9 Pregnancy/postpartum
10 Prolonged or traumatic CPR
11 Bleeding disorders or anticoagulation with INR > 1.8
12 Probable intracardiac thrombus
13 Cerebral infarct within the last three months (controversial)

14 Current menstrual bleeding.

HEART FAILURE

Causes of heart failure

1 IHD
2 Arrhythmia
3 Valvular or congenital heart disease
4 Drugs:
    (a) negative inotropes, e.g. beta-blockers
    (b) drugs with fluid-retaining properties, e.g. steroids, NSAIDs
5 Myocarditis or pericarditis
6 Cardiomyopathy
7 Increased metabolic demand:
    (a) pregnancy
    (b) hyperthyroidism
    (c) anaemia
8 PE
9 Intercurrent illness
10 Inappropriate reduction of therapy.

Complications of heart failure

1 Uraemia
2 Electrolyte disturbance:
    (a) hypokalaemia
    (b) hyponatraemia
3 Liver impairment
4 Thromboembolism:
    (a) DVT/PE
    (b) systemic (due to AF or intracardiac thrombus)
5 Arrhythmias:
    (a) atrial or ventricular
    (b) may be drug-related
    (c) may cause up to 50% of deaths in patients with cardiac failure
6 Weight loss.

Treatments for heart failure

1 Low salt diet
2 Fluid restriction
3 Loop Diuretics
4 Thiazide diuretics
5 ACE inhibitors
6 Beta-blockers (bisoprolol, carvedilol and metoprolol)
7 Spironolactone
8 Digoxin
9 Nitrates
10 Hydralazine
11 Anticoagulation
12 Ionotropes
13 Cardiac transplantation.

HYPERTENSION (see also page 295)

Causes of systemic hypertension

1 Primary/idiopathic/essential hypertension
2 Renal disease:
   (a) renal artery stenosis
   (b) polycystic kidney disease
   (c) renal parenchymal disease (e.g. glomerulonephritis)
   (d) chronic renal failure
3 Coarctation of the aorta
4 Endocrine disease:
   (a) diabetes mellitus
   (b) phaeochromocytoma
   (c) Conn's syndrome (primary hyperaldosteronism)
   (d) Cushing's syndrome
   (e) acromegaly
   (f) hyperparathyroidism
   (g) congenital adrenal hyperplasia
5 Drugs:
   (a) steroids (corticosteroids, anabolic steroids, oestrogen-containing oral contraceptives)
   (b) NSAIDs

   (c) sympathomimetics
6 Pregnancy
   (a) pre-eclampsia
   (b) eclampsia
7 Neurogenic
   (a) post head injury
   (b) post stroke.

Complications of systemic hypertension

1 CVA – haemorrhage or infarct
2 Retinopathy
3 Left ventricular hypertrophy/failure
4 IHD
5 Aortic aneurysm plus PVD
6 Renal impairment
7 Increased frequency of subarachnoid haemorrhage
8 Hypertensive encephalopathy (rare).

VALVULAR HEART DISEASE

Causes of mitral stenosis

1 Rheumatic fever
2 Congenital
3 Carcinoid syndrome
4 SLE
5 Mucopolysaccharide disorders
6 Viral myocarditis.

Causes of mitral regurgitation

  1 'Functional', due to LV impairment
  2 Rheumatic fever
  3 Mitral valve prolapse
  4 Collagen disorders (e.g. Marfan's syndrome)
  5 IHD:
     (a) post MI
     (b) papillary muscle ischaemia
  6 Endocarditis/myocarditis

7 Connective tissue disorders (e.g. SLE)
8 Idiopathic
9 Associated with congenital heart defects (e.g. ASD)
10 Cardiomyopathy.

Associations with mitral valve prolapse

1 IHD
2 Cardiomyopathy
3 Congenital heart defects:
   (a) PDA
   (b) ostium secundum ASD
4 Wolff–Parkinson–White syndrome
5 Myocarditis
6 Connective tissue and collagen disorders:
   (a) Marfan's syndrome
   (b) pseudoxanthoma elastica
   (c) osteogenesis imperfecta
   (d) SLE
   (e) PAN
7 Left atrial myxoma
8 Muscular dystrophy
9 Polycystic kidney disease.

Causes of aortic stenosis

Stenosis of the aortic valve itself may be caused by:
1 Congenital aortic stenosis
2 Congenitally bicuspid valve (more common in men)
3 Degenerative calcification (more common in women)
4 Rheumatic fever.

Subvalvular stenosis

1 Congenital
2 Hypertrophic cardiomyopathy
3 Subaortic membranous stenosis.

Supravalvular stenosis

1 Congenital

2 Coarctation of the aorta
3 Williams syndrome.

Causes of aortic regurgitation

1 Congenital – bicuspid or other form of abnormal valve
2 Inflammatory conditions:
    (a) rheumatic fever
    (b) infective endocarditis
    (c) rheumatoid arthritis
    (d) SLE
3 Aortic dilatation:
    (a) Marfan's syndrome
    (b) syphilis
    (c) ankylosing spondylitis and other seronegative arthropathies
    (d) atheroma
4 Collagen disorders:
    (a) Marfan's syndrome
    (b) Hurler's syndrome
    (c) pseudoxanthoma elastica
5 Aortic dissection
6 Trauma
7 Hypertension
8 VSD with prolapsed right coronary cusp
9 Ruptured sinus of Valsalva aneurysm.

Causes of tricuspid regurgitation

1 'Functional', due to RV dilatation resulting from pulmonary hypertension or cor pulmonale
2 Right ventricular infarction
3 Rheumatic fever
4 Infective endocarditis (particularly in intravenous drug users)
5 Carcinoid syndrome
6 Ebstein's anomaly (a congenitally malpositioned tricuspid valve).

Causes of pulmonary stenosis

1 Congenital
2 Carcinoid syndrome (a late sign).

Infective endocarditis

Predisposing factors

1 Rheumatic heart disease
2 Degenerative heart disease
3 Mitral valve prolapse
4 Congenital heart disease (bicuspid aortic valve is most common)
5 Hypertrophic cardiomyopathy
6 Intravenous drug use
7 Prosthetic valves.

Microbiology

1 Viridans steptococci
2 Streptococcus bovis
3 Staphylococcus aureus
4 Enterococci
5 Haemophilus spp.
6 Streptococcus pneumoniae
7 Cardiobacterium hominis
8 Gram negative
9 Coxiella burnetii.

Clinical features

1 Fever (90%)
2 Anorexia and weight loss
3 New or changing murmur
4 Splinter haemorrhages
5 Petechiae
6 Osler's nodes
7 Janeway lesions
8 Roth spots
9 Systemic emboli
10 Mycotic aneurysms.

CONGENITAL HEART DISEASE

Causes of cyanotic congenital heart disease

Right-to-left shunt:
1 Tetralogy of Fallot
2 Complete transposition of the great vessels
3 Severe Ebstein's anomaly
Without a shunt:
4 Tricuspid atresia
5 Pulmonary atresia
6 Severe pulmonary stenosis
7 Hypoplastic left heart
Reversal of a previous left-to-right shunt:
8 Eisenmenger's syndrome.

Causes of acyanotic congenital heart disease

Left-to-right shunt:
1 Coarctation of the aorta associated with VSD or PDA
2 Ventricular septal defect
3 Atrial septal defect
4 Patent ductus arteriosus
5 Partial anomalous pulmonary venous drainage
Without a shunt:
6 Congenital aortic stenosis
7 Coarctation of the aorta without VSD or PDA.

Atrial septal defect (ASD)

ASD accounts for 10% of congenital heart disease.

Ostium secundum (70%)

1 Defect of fossa ovale
2 Associated with MVP (mitral valve prolapse)
3 Partial RBBB with RAD on ECG
4 20% develop AF later in life
5 Low risk of endocarditis.

Ostium primum (15%)

1 Usually detected earlier in childhood
2 Associated with MR
3 ECG shows RBBB, LAD and first-degree block
4 Associated with Down's, Klinefelter's and Noonan's syndromes.

Sinus venosus (15%)

1 Defect in upper part of septum
2 Often associated with anomalous pulmonary venous drainage.

Clinical features

1 Wide fixed splitting of the second heart sound
2 Pulmonary flow murmur (systolic)
3 Tricuspid diastolic murmur if shunt is large.

CXR

1 Cardiac enlargement
2 Enlarged pulmonary artery
3 Pulmonary plethora.

Complications

1 AF
2 Eisenmenger's syndrome (reversal of the left-to-right shunt due
   to development of pulmonary hypertension)
3 Tricuspid regurgitation
4 Cardiac failure (if defect is large)
5 Infective endocarditis (rarely).

Ventricular septal defect (VSD)

Accounts for 25–30% of congenital heart defects; 30–50% close
spontaneously. Defects may be:
1 Muscular
2 Membranous
3 Atrio-ventricular
4 Infundibular
5 Into right atrium (Gerbode defect).

Maladie de Roger is a small defect associated with loud murmur.

Clinical features

1 Pansystolic murmur throughout precordium but loudest at LSE
2 Parasternal thrill
3 Single S2 may be heard if defect is large (absent A2)
4 Diastolic mitral murmur (if defect is large).

Cardiac associations

1 PDA
2 Aortic regurgitation
3 Pulmonary stenosis
4 ASD
5 Tetralogy of Fallot
6 Coarctation of the aorta.

Complications

1 Subacute bacterial endocarditis
2 Eisenmenger's syndrome
3 Cardiac failure.

Patent ductus arteriosus (PDA)

Accounts for 15% of congenital heart disease; commoner in females. Associated with maternal rubella. May be closed with indometacin, or kept open with prostaglandins (used when associated with some cyanotic congenital heart disorders prior to corrective surgery).

Clinical features

1 Collapsing pulse
2 LVH
3 Continuous machinery murmur (maximal 2nd LICS and posteriorly)
4 Left subclavicular thrill.

Complications

1 'Endocarditis' of the ductus

2 Eisenmenger's syndrome.

Tetralogy of Fallot

Forms 10% of cyanotic congenital heart disease. Usually presents after six months of age. It has four components:
1 Pulmonary stenosis
2 Right ventricular hypertrophy
3 VSD (right-to-left shunt due to the pulmonary stenosis)
4 Overriding of the VSD by the aorta.

Clinical features

1 Cyanotic attacks (due to pulmonary infundibular spasm) with syncope (children often squat in an effort to reduce these)
2 Clubbing
3 Parasternal heave
4 Ejection systolic murmur in pulmonary area
5 Systolic thrill
6 Quiet or inaudible P2
7 RVH on ECG.

CXR

1 Boot-shaped heart (normal size)
2 Small pulmonary artery
3 Large aorta
4 Pulmonary oligaemia.

Complications

1 Cerebral abscesses (10%)
2 Endocarditis (10%)
3 Paradoxical embolus
4 Polycythaemia
5 Coagulopathy
6 Ventricular arrhythmias.

Coarctation of the aorta

Accounts for 5% of congenital heart disease, more common in males.

Most are distal to the origin of the left subclavian artery. Rarely, may be acquired later in life (e.g. due to progressive arteritis – Takayasu's disease – or trauma).

Associations

1 Berry aneurysms
2 Turner's syndrome
3 Renal abnormalities
4 Bicuspid aortic valve
5 PDA
6 VSD
7 Mitral valve disease.

Clinical features

1 May be asymptomatic
2 Hypertension in upper part of the body (may cause headaches and nose bleeds)
3 Radiofemoral delay
4 Absent or weak femoral pulses
5 Systolic murmur (infraclavicular or posterior)
6 Collateral artery formation (around scapulae or below ribs posteriorly)
7 LVH on ECG.

CXR

1 Double aortic knuckle.
2 Rib notching.

Complications

1 Headaches
2 CVA
3 Left ventricular failure
4 Endocarditis
5 Premature IHD
6 Aortic dissection.

Eisenmenger's syndrome

Reversal of left-to-right shunt due to development of pulmonary hypertension. Occurs in VSD, ASD and PDA.

Clinical features

1 Decreasing intensity of murmurs
2 Single S2
3 Louder, palpable P2
4 Right ventricular heave
5 Graham Steell murmur (pulmonary regurgitation)
6 V waves in JVP (due to TR, which may be associated with a murmur)
7 Central cyanosis
8 Clubbing.

ECG

Shows signs of RVH.

CXR

1 Enlarged pulmonary vessels
2 Peripheral pruning.

Complications

1 Heart failure (cor pulmonale)
2 Syncope
3 Angina
4 Massive haemoptysis
5 Cerebral abscess or embolus
6 Infective endocarditis (rare).

Clinical Pharmacology

DRUG METABOLISM AND PHARMACOKINETICS

Important liver enzyme inducers

Inducers of cytochrome P450, > 200 known.
PC BRASS:
1 **P** henytoin
2 **C** arbamazepine
3 **B** arbiturates
4 **R** ifampicin
5 **A** lcohol (chronic use)
6 **S** ulphonylureas
7 **S** moking.

Important drugs whose metabolism is affected by enzyme inducers

Drugs metabolised by cytochrome P450 – leads to **increased** metabolism of the drug:
1 Warfarin ($\downarrow$ INR)
2 OCP (pregnancy)
3 Corticosteroids ($\downarrow$ effect)
4 Ciclosporin ($\downarrow$ immunosuppression)
5 Theophyllines ($\downarrow$ effect)
6 All of the enzyme inducers themselves ($\downarrow$ effect).

45

Important liver enzyme inhibitors

These drugs lead to **reduced** metabolism of the drug and toxicity.
OAAK DEVVICCES:
1 **O** meprazole
2 **A** miodarone
3 **A** llopurinol
4 **K** etoconazole (and fluconazole)
5 **D** isulfiram
6 **E** rythromycin
7 **V** alproate
8 **V** erapamil
9 **I** soniazid
10 **C** iprofloxacin
11 **C** imetidine
12 **E** thanol (acute)
13 **S** ulphonamides.

Important drugs affected by liver enzyme inhibitors

1 Warfarin ($\uparrow$ INR)
2 Phenytoin (toxicity)
3 Carbamazepine (toxicity)
4 Theophylline (toxicity)
5 Ciclosporin (toxicity).

Clinically important drug interactions

[See Table 1, opposite]

Drugs exhibiting zero-order kinetics (saturation kinetics)

1 Alcohol
2 Phenytoin
3 Fluoxetine.

Drugs exhibiting partial agonist activity

1 Oxprenolol
2 Buprenorphine
3 Methysergide
4 Tamoxifen
5 Pentazocine.

Table 1

Drug I	Drug II	Effect
Azathioprine Mercaptopurine	Allopurinol	Xanthine oxidase inhibition leads to azathioprine toxicity
	Cyclophosphamide	Reduced clearance of cyclophosphamide leading to ↑ toxicity
Alcohol	Metronidazole Chlorpropamide	Flushing, hypotension
MAOIs	Tyramine Alpha-agonists Amphetamines	Acute hypertensive crisis
	Pethidine	CNS excitation
ACE inhibitors	K-sparing diuretics	Hyperkalaemia
	NSAIDs	Reduced effect of ACE inhibitors
Digoxin	Thiazides Loop diuretics Amiodarone Nifedipine Verapamil	Digoxin toxicity by ↓ protein binding/renal excretion
	Antacids Cholestyramine	↓ Absorption
Beta-blockers	Verapamil	Hypotension and asystole
Lithium	Thiazides	Lithium toxicity (↓ excretion)
Adenosine	Dipyridamole	Prolonged half-life of adenosine leading to asystole
Statins	Fibrates Ciclosporin	Increased incidence of myopathy and rhabdomyolysis
Aminoglycosides	Loop diuretics	Increased nephrotoxicity and ototoxicity

Pro-drugs

Examples of drugs that need to be metabolised before having an effect:

1 Enalapril
2 Azathioprine
3 L-dopa
4 Aciclovir
5 Spironolactone
6 Zidovudine (AZT)
7 Cyclophosphamide.

Drugs that cause their effect by inhibiting enzymes

Table 2

Drug	Enzyme inhibited
ACE inhibitors	Angiotensin-converting enzyme
Aciclovir	DNA polymerase
Allopurinol	Xanthine oxidase
Zidovudine (AZT)	Reverse transcriptase
Disulfiram	Aldehyde dehydrogenase
MAOIs	Monoamine oxidase
Methotrexate/trimethoprim	Dihydrofolate reductase
Neostigmine	Cholinesterases
Aspirin/NSAIDs	Cyclo-oxygenase (COX)
Penicillins	Transpeptidase
Vigabatrin	GABA transaminase

Drugs for which therapeutic monitoring is useful

These are drugs that show good correlation between blood concentration and therapeutic effect.

1 Digoxin
2 Lithium
3 Aminoglycosides
4 Vancomycin
5 Phenytoin
6 Carbamazepine
7 Theophylline
8 Ciclosporin
9 Phenobarbital.

Drugs in the elderly

1 Gastric pH ↑, gastric emptying ↓, ↓ blood flow – affects absorption of drugs
2 Absorption from intramuscular injections slower due to ↓ muscle mass and ↓ blood flow to muscles
3 Reduced hepatic extraction and metabolism
4 Half-life of some drugs prolonged (e.g. benzodiazepines)
5 Greater volume of fat leads to increased volume of distribution for lipid-soluble drugs

6 GFR reduced in the elderly, leading to accumulation of renally excreted drugs (lithium, digoxin etc.)
7 Changes in homeostatic responses make the elderly more susceptible to side-effects of some drugs
8 Polypharmacy leads to more interactions.

Drugs and the kidney

Drugs causing direct nephrotoxicity

Generally avoid these drugs in renal impairment unless there is a specific indication, e.g. ACE inhibitors.
1 *Glomerular damage:*
   (a) penicillamine
   (b) gold
   (c) captopril
2 *Alteration of renal vascular dynamics:*
   (a) ACE inhibitors
   (b) NSAIDs
   (c) ciclosporin
3 *Tubular damage:*
   (a) amphotericin
   (b) aminoglycosides
   (c) cisplatin
   (d) demeclocycline
   (e) lithium
   (f) thiazides
4 *Interstitial damage:*
   (a) NSAIDs
   (b) sulphonamides
   (c) 5-ASA drugs
   (d) vancomycin.

Drugs excreted unchanged by the kidney

1 Atenolol
2 Antibiotics:
   (a) penicillins
   (b) cephalosporins
   (c) aminoglycosides
   (d) tetracycline

3 Furosemide (frusemide)
4 Thiazides
5 Digoxin
6 Lithium
7 Chlorpropamide
8 Metformin
9 H₂ blockers
10 Aspirin (in overdose).

Drugs to use with caution or in reduced dosage in renal failure

1 Aciclovir
2 ACE inhibitors
3 Aminoglycosides
4 Allopurinol
5 Cephalosporins
6 Digoxin
7 H₂ blockers
8 Penicillins
9 Sulphonylureas
10 Vigabatrin.

Drugs to avoid in renal failure

1 Chlorpropamide
2 Retinoids
3 Metformin
4 Nitrofurantoin
5 Methotrexate
6 Tetracyclines
7 Amphotericin
8 NSAIDs
9 Lithium
10 Gold
11 Penicllamine
12 Vancomycin.

Drugs and the liver

Drugs which undergo major hepatic metabolism

1 Beta-blockers:

(a) propranolol
(b) labetolol
(c) metoprolol
2 Beta-agonists:
   (a) salbutamol
   (b) terbutaline
3 Rifampicin
4 Erythromycin
5 Spironolactone
6 Cardiac drugs:
   (a) GTN
   (b) verapamil
   (c) nifedipine
   (d) lidocaine (lignocaine)
   (e) digitoxin (cf. digoxin)
   (f) prazosin
7 CNS drugs:
   (a) chlormethiazole
   (b) tricyclic antidepressants
   (c) phenothiazines
   (d) benzodiazepines
   (e) barbiturates
   (f) L-dopa
8 Analgesics:
   (a) paracetamol
   (b) pethidine
   (c) aspirin.

Drugs which cause jaundice – see Gastroenterology
(see also pages 160–161)

Genetic polymorphisms determining drug toxicity

Essential features of acetylator status

Toxic effects of some drugs depend on speed of acetylation and metabolism. There are slow acetylators (incidence 50%) and fast acetylators – genetically determined.

Table 3

	Slow	Fast (increased toxic metabolites)
Isoniazid	Neuropathy (glove and stocking) Drug-induced SLE ↑ Phenytoin toxicity ↑ Carbamazepine toxicity ↑ Rifampicin	Failure of TB therapy Hepatitis
Sulfasalazine	↑ Toxicity (headaches, leucopenia) ↑ Haemolysis in G6PD-deficient patients	
Hydralazine	Drug-induced SLE	↓ BP control
Procainamide	Drug-induced SLE	
Dapsone	↑ Haemolysis in G6PD-deficient patients	↓ Benefit in dermatitis herpetiformis

Diseases associated with slow acetylator status:
1 Gilbert's syndrome
2 Sjögren's syndrome
3 Arylamine-induced bladder cancer.

Essential features of G6PD deficiency (see also page 188)

1 X-linked dominant inheritance
2 Present in 5–10% of black males
3 Predisposes to haemolytic anaemia
4 Heterozygotes demonstrate increased resistance to malaria
5 Drugs causing haemolysis in these patients:
   (a) primaquine
   (b) sulphonamides
   (c) sulfasalazine
   (d) dapsone
   (e) quinolones (e.g. ciprofloxacin)
   (f) nitrofurantoin
   (g) nalidixic acid.

Other drugs causing haemolytic anaemia (immune-mediated)

1 Penicillins

2 Methyldopa
3 Quinine
4 Quinidine
5 Sulphonylureas.

Important drugs that precipitate acute attacks of porphyria
(see also page 263)

1 All enzyme inducers (see above)
2 ACE inhibitors
3 Erythromycin
4 Sulphonamides
5 Furosemide (frusemide)
6 OCP
7 Calcium channel blockers.

Some drugs that are safe in porphyria

1 Aspirin
2 Beta-blockers
3 Penicillin
4 Morphine + codeine
5 Paracetamol
6 Metformin.

Other genetic polymorphisms

Table 4

Polymorphism	Toxicity
Pseudocholinesterase deficiency (AR)	Suxamethonium toxicity, prolonged apnoea post-anaesthesia
Malignant hyperthermia (AD)	Hypercatabolic response to halothane, suxamethonium, tricyclics, MAOIs
Steroid-induced glaucoma (AR)	5% population
Sulphonylurea flushing (AD)	30% population
Warfarin resistance (AD)	Rare
Cytochrome P450 polymorphisms	Leads to altered metabolism
e.g. omeprazole	2% population
nortriptyline	10% population
metoprolol	10% population

Drugs in pregnancy and breastfeeding

Physiological changes affecting drug metabolism

1 ↑ GFR
2 ↑ Metabolism by P450 enzymes (induction)
3 ↑ Volume of distribution
4 ↓ Protein binding
5 ↓ Gastric emptying.

Drugs causing teratogenesis (first trimester)

Table 5

Agent	Effect
Thalidomide	Phocomelia, heart defects
Anticonvulsants:	
Carbamazepine	Neural tube defects
Phenytoin	Cleft palate, microcephaly, retardation
Valproate	Neural tube defects
Cytotoxics (including folic acid antagonists)	Hydrocephalus, neural tube defects, cleft palate
Alcohol	Fetal alcohol syndrome
Warfarin	Retarded growth, limb defects, saddle nose
Diethylstilbestrol	Adenocarcinoma of vagina (20 years later)
Oestrogens	Testicular atrophy in males
Anabolic steroids	Masculinisation in females
ACE inhibitors	Oligohydramnios, renal failure
Retinoids	Hydrocephalus, neural tube defects
Lithium	Heart defects

Drugs affecting the fetus during intrauterine life and the neonatal period

Table 6

Drug	Effect
Antibiotics	
Tetracyclines	Tooth discoloration
Aminoglycosides	VIII cranial nerve damage
Sulphonamides	Jaundice, kernicterus, neonatal haemolysis and methaemoglobinaemia
Chloramphenicol	Cardiovascular collapse of the newborn ('grey baby syndrome')
Antithyroid drugs	
Iodides	Neonatal hypothyroidism, goitre
Carbimazole	
Anticoagulants	
Warfarin	Fetal and neonatal haemorrhage
Hypoglycaemics	
Sulphonylureas	Fetal and neonatal hypoglycaemia
Cardiovascular drugs	
Beta-agonists	Fetal tachycardia, delayed labour
Beta-antagonists	Fetal and neonatal bradycardia, neonatal hypoglycaemia, IUGR
CNS drugs	
Alcohol	CNS depression, withdrawal syndromes
Barbituates	
Narcotics	
Benzodiazepines	
Lithium	Neonatal hypothyroidism, goitre
Corticosteroids and sex hormones	Fetal and neonatal adrenal suppression, virilisation of female fetus
NSAIDs	
Aspirin	Premature closure of ductus arteriosus, delayed labour, increased blood loss, impaired platelet function
Indometacin	

Drugs contraindicated in breastfeeding

1 Amiodarone (thyroid anomalies)
2 Aspirin (Reye's syndrome, hypoprothrombinaemia, impaired platelet function)

3 Indometacin (seizures)
4 ACE inhibitors
5 Cytotoxics
6 Benzodiazepines (sedation, respiratory depression)
7 Ergotamine (ergotism)
8 Lithium (involuntary movements)
9 Phenytoin
10 Retinoids
11 Sex hormones (feminisation of males, masculinisation of females)
12 Tetracyclines (tooth discoloration)
13 Gold (renal impairment, haematological reactions)
14 Vitamin A (toxicity)
15 Vitamin D (hypercalcaemia).

Drugs that are relatively safe in pregnancy

1 Heparin
2 Insulin
3 Thyroxine
4 Antibiotics:
    (a) penicillins
    (b) cephalosporins
    (c) erythromycin
    (d) ethambutol
    (e) isoniazid
5 Inhaled salbutamol
6 Methyldopa
7 Hydralazine
8 Paracetamol
9 Metoclopramide
10 Cyclizine.

DRUG SIDE-EFFECTS

Peripheral neuropathy

1 Tricyclic antidepressants
2 Amiodarone
3 Metronidazole

4 Nitrofurantoin
5 Zidovudine
6 Vinka alkaloids
7 Isoniazid (use pyridoxine for prevention)
8 Phenytoin.

Drugs that cause convulsions

1 Penicillins
2 Ciprofloxacin
3 Chlorpromazine
4 TCAs (tricyclic antidepressants)
5 Halothane
6 Lidocaine (lignocaine)
7 Intravenous contrast media
8 Pethidine
9 Lithium
10 Cimetidine
11 Chloroquine
12 All antiepileptics.

Drugs that cause agranulocytosis/neutropenia

1 Carbimazole
2 Zidovudine (AZT)
3 Clozapine
4 Mianserin
5 NSAIDs
6 Sulphonylureas
7 Sulphonamides
8 Cytotoxics
9 Captopril
10 Cephalosporins
11 Chloramphenicol
12 Dapsone
13 Penicillins.

Drugs that cause gum hypertrophy

1 Phenytoin
2 Nifedipine

3 Ciclosporin.

Gum hypertrophy may also occur in scurvy, pregnancy and in acute promyelocytic leukaemia.

Drugs that cause gynaecomastia

1 Cimetidine
2 Cyproterone
3 Digoxin
4 Oestrogens
5 Spironolactone
6 Ketoconazole
7 Phenothiazines.

Drugs that cause bronchoconstriction

1 Adenosine
2 Beta-blockers
3 NSAIDs
4 ACE inhibitors
5 Muscle relaxants
6 Some opioids.

Drugs that cause pulmonary oedema

1 Adrenaline (epinephrine)
2 Diamorphine
3 Thiazides
4 Intravenous fluids
5 Intravenous beta blockers
6 Methadone
7 Naloxone
8 Salicylate overdose
9 Tricyclic antidepressant overdose.

Drugs that cause pulmonary eosinophilia

1 Carbamazepine
2 Phenytoin
3 Sulphonamides

4 Dantrolene
5 Nitrofurantoin
6 Penicillin
7 Erythromycin
8 Chlorpropamide.

Drugs that cause syndrome of inappropriate antidiuretic hormone secretion (SIADH)

1 Opiates
2 Carbamazepine
3 Oxytocin
4 Chlorpropamide
5 Phenothiazines
6 Tricyclic antidepressants
7 Cytotoxics (vincristine, cyclophosphamide)
8 Rifampicin
9 Drugs that precipitate porphyria.

Drugs that cause nephrogenic diabetes insipidus

1 Lithium
2 Demeclocycline (used to treat SIADH)
3 Amphotericin
4 Glibenclamide.

For extra-pyramidal side-effects, see Neurology; drugs causing gout, see Rheumatology; drugs that cause pulmonary fibrosis, see Respiratory medicine; drugs causing photosensitivity, see Dermatology; and drugs causing hyperprolactinaemia, see Endocrinology.

FEATURES OF DRUGS THAT APPEAR COMMONLY IN EXAMS

Amiodarone

1 Increases the refractory period of cardiac muscle (Class III effect)
2 Effective for both atrial and ventricular arrhythmias
3 *Indications:*
   (a) AF treatment and prophylaxis

    (b) WPW syndrome
    (c) VT treatment and prophylaxis
    (d) HCM
4 Very long half-life (10–100 days) so accumulates in organs
5 Not negatively inotropic
6 Prolongs survival in HCM ($\downarrow$ fatal arrhythmias)
7 *Side-effects:*
    (a) photosensitive rash
    (b) slate-grey skin pigmentation (deposition in the skin)
    (c) hypothyroidism (more common than hyper-):
        $\uparrow$ production of reverse T3 in liver
    (d) hyperthyoidism: $\uparrow$ T4$\rightarrow$T3
    (e) alveolitis
    (f) peripheral neuropathy
    (g) ataxia
    (h) metallic taste
    (i) hepatitis
    (j) corneal microdeposits (reversible and not clinically significant)
    (k) torsades de pointes arrhythmias (prolongs QT interval).

Digoxin

1 Cardiac glycoside
2 Acts at Na/K-ATPase leading to inhibition of Na/K pump
3 Slows conduction through the AV node leading to rate control in AF
   (will not cardiovert)
4 $\uparrow$ Vagal tone
5 Positively inotropic
6 Renal excretion
7 Several interactions (see Table 1, page 41)
8 Severe overdose treated with digoxin-specific antibody fragments
   (Digibind®)
9 *Indications:*
    (a) rate control in AF
    (b) CCF
10 *Contraindications:*
    (a) CHB
    (b) 2nd degree AV block
    (c) WPW syndrome
    (d) HCM

11 *Adverse effects:*
  (a) any arrhythmia (SVT most common)
  (b) nausea and vomiting
  (c) diarrhoea
  (d) confusion and headache
  (e) gynaecomastia
  (f) visual disturbance
12 Toxicity enhanced by:
  (a) ↓ K
  (b) ↓ Mg
  (c) ↑ Ca
  (d) hypothyroidism
  (e) ↓ GFR
  (f) ↑ age.

Thiazides

1 Act at the distal convoluted tubule
2 Inhibit Na/Cl cotransporter reducing reabsorption of NaCl
3 *Indications:*
  (a) hypertension
  (b) heart failure
  (c) prevention of recurrent renal stone formation in idiopathic hypercalciuria
  (d) nephrogenic diabetes insipidus
4 *Adverse effects:*
  (a) hypokalaemia
  (b) hyponatraemia
  (c) hypercalcaemia
  (d) hyperuricaemia
  (e) hypomagnesaemia
  (f) hypochloraemic alkalosis
  (g) hyperglycaemia
  (h) hypercholesterolaemia
  (i) impotence
  (j) postural hypotension.

ACE inhibitors

1 Inhibit the conversion of angiotensin I to angiotensin II

2 *Indications:*
   (a) hypertension
   (b) heart failure (↓ mortality in all grades)
   (c) post MI, particularly with ventricular dysfunction (↓ mortality)
   (d) diabetic nephropathy even if BP normal (↓ proteinuria and deterioration in renal function)
   (e) susceptible patients over 55 years – prevention of MI, stroke or cardiovascular death
3 *Contraindications:*
   (a) bilateral renal artery stenosis – leads to renal failure due to ↓ GFR
   (b) hereditary angio-oedema
   (c) aortic stenosis
   (d) pregnancy
4 *Adverse effects:*
   (a) renal impairment
   (b) hypotension (more severe in those on high-dose diuretics)
   (c) hyperkalaemia
   (d) proteinuria
   (e) nephrotic syndrome
   (f) neutropenia and agranulocytosis
   (g) rash
   (h) photosensitivity
   (i) alteration of taste
   (j) cough (due to the inhibition of bradykinin metabolism in the lungs)
   (k) angio-oedema
   (l) abnormal LFTs (cholestasis and hepatitis).

Angiotensin II inhibitors

1 Do not inhibit bradykinin metabolism so do not cause cough
2 Use with care in renal artery stenosis – can lead to renal failure
3 Can cause angio-oedema
4 Avoid in pregnancy
5 Currently only licensed for use in hypertension.

Phenytoin

1 Voltage-activated Na blocker – stabilises membrane
2 Zero-order kinetics

3 Enzyme inducer
4 Useful for partial and generalised seizures but not absence
5 *Toxic effects:*
   (a) ataxia
   (b) nystagmus
   (c) vertigo
   (d) tremor
   (e) dysarthria
   (f) coma
   (g) arrhythmias
6 *Side-effects:*
   (a) gum hypertrophy
   (b) hirsutism
   (c) megaloblastic anaemia
   (d) seizures
   (e) coarse facies
   (f) osteomalacia
   (g) lupus
   (h) erythema nodosum
   (i) hepatitis
   (j) Dupuytren's contracture
   (k) IgA deficiency.

Ciclosporin

1 Powerful immunosuppressive which inhibits lymphocytes
2 Affects cell-mediated and antibody-mediated reactions
3 Main effect is inhibition cytotoxic T cells via IL-2
4 Does not cause bone marrow suppression
5 *Indications:*
   (a) transplant rejection
   (b) RA
   (c) psoriasis
   (d) atopic dermatitis
6 *Adverse effects:*
   (a) nephrotoxicity
   (b) hypertension
   (c) gum hypertrophy
   (d) hepatotoxicity
   (e) tremor

(f) paraesthesiae of hands and feet
(g) hypertrichosis
(h) increased risk of skin cancers and lymphoproliferative malignancies.

Chlorpromazine (phenothiazines)

1 Neuroleptic drug
2 Blocks dopamine (D2), alpha, muscarinic and histamine receptors
3 *Side-effects:*
   (a) sedation
   (b) hypothermia
   (c) cholestatic jaundice
   (d) anticholinergic effects (dry mouth etc.)
   (e) photosensitivity
   (f) postural hypotension
   (g) agranulocytosis
   (h) prolonged QT (leading to VT)
   (i) dystonia
   (j) neuroleptic malignant syndrome
   (k) extrapyramidal effects (can be reduced by administration of antimuscarinic drugs)
   (l) oculogyric crisis
   (m) tardive dyskinesia
   (n) akathisia
   (o) hyperprolactinaemia (may lead to gynaecomastia).

Clozapine

1 Atypical neuroleptic
2 Dopamine receptor antagonists (particularly D4)
3 More efficacious than chlorpromazine
4 Fewer extrapyramidal side-effects than chlorpromazine
5 Causes agranulocytosis in 1% of patients
6 Causes convulsions in 3% of patients.

Lithium

1 Used for prophylaxis of bipolar affective disorder, treatment of mania and prophylaxis of recurrent depression
2 Narrow therapeutic index so monitoring important (therapeutic serum

level 0.5–1.0 mmol/l)
3 Toxicity more likely in renal impairment
4 *Lithium excretion reduced by:*
   (a) thiazides
   (b) loop diuretics
   (c) ACE inhibitors
   (d) NSAIDs
5 *Adverse effects:*
   (a) tremor (15%)
   (b) weight gain and oedema
   (c) thirst and polyuria
   (d) nausea, vomiting and diarrhoea
   (e) nephrogenic diabetes insipidus
   (f) hypothyroidism
   (g) interstitial nephritis
   (h) teratogenicity
   (i) confusion
6 *Overdosage (> 1.5 mmol/l):*
   (a) tremor
   (b) ataxia
   (c) dysarthria
   (d) nystagmus
   (e) renal impairment
   (f) convulsions
7 *Overdosage (> 2 mmol/l):*
   (a) above +
   (b) hyperreflexia
   (c) toxic psychosis
   (d) oliguria
   (e) circulatory failure
   (f) coma
   (g) death
8 *Treatment of overdose:*
   (a) stop lithium
   (b) stop diuretics and NSAIDs
   (c) gastric lavage (within 6–8 hours)
   (d) forced diuresis
   (e) haemodialysis.

Retinoids

1 Vitamin A derivatives
2 *Indications:*
   (a) psoriasis
   (b) acne
   (c) acute promyelocytic leukaemia
3 *Side-effects:*
   (a) mucosal dryness
   (b) alopecia
   (c) hypertriglyceridaemia
   (d) thrombocytopenia
   (e) reduced night vision
   (f) photosensitivity
   (g) mood changes
   (h) hepatitis
   (i) teratogenicity
   (j) benign intracranial hypertension
   (k) skeletal hyperostosis (high doses).

Tamoxifen

1 Anti-oestrogen drug used for oestrogen-positive breast tumours
2 60% of oestrogen receptor +ve respond; 10% of oestrogen receptor −ve respond
3 Partial agonist
4 Delays metastases and prolongs survival
5 Should be continued for five years
6 *Adverse effects:*
   (a) tumour flare
   (b) hypercalcaemia
   (c) amenorrhoea
   (d) hot flushes
   (e) endometrial hyperplasia and cancer
   (f) alopecia
   (g) leucopenia
   (h) visual disturbance.

Carbimazole

1 Inhibits peroxidase therefore reducing iodination of tyrosil residues on thyroglobulin

2 May have immunological modulatory properties that cause remission of Graves' disease
3 Takes several weeks to work
4 Crosses the placenta and is present in breast milk
5 *Adverse effects:*
   (a) agranulocytosis (reversible on stopping the drug)
   (b) rashes common (up to 25%)
   (c) arthralgia
   (d) jaundice
   (e) nausea and vomiting.

Interferons

1 *Indications:*
   (a) *alpha:*
      (i) hepatitis B (chronic)
      (ii) hepatitis C (chronic)
      (iii) hairy cell leukaemia
      (iv) AIDS-related Kaposi's sarcoma
      (v) condylomata acuminata
      (vi) renal cell carcinoma
      (vii) CML
      (viii) some lymphomas
   (b) *beta:*
      (i) MS
   (c) *gamma:*
      (i) reduction of risk of infection in chronic granulomatous disease
2 *Side-effects:*
   (a) nausea
   (b) influenza-like symptoms
   (c) lethargy
   (d) depression
   (e) hypersensitivity
   (f) myelosuppression.

NEWER DRUGS

Tumour necrosis factor-alpha (TNF-α) antagonists

1 Infliximab (chimeric IgG monoclonal antibody which inhibits TNF-α)
2 Etanercept (recombinant molecule that inactivates TNF-α and -β)

3 *Indications:*
   (a) RA (severe)
   (b) juvenile chronic arthritis
   (c) Crohn's disease (severe, unresponsive to conventional therapy)
   (d) Crohn's fistulae
4 *Adverse effects:*
   (a) infusion-related effects (fever, pruritus, urticaria, hypotension)
   (b) ANA or ds DNA antibodies develop in some patients
   (c) drug-induced lupus
   (d) infections
   (e) reactivation of TB
   (f) leucopenia
   (g) avoid in pregnancy and breastfeeding.

Granulocyte macrophage colony-stimulating factor (GM-CSF)

1 Haematopoetic growth factor
2 Enhances survival of cells committed to the granulocytic and macrophage lineages and stimulates their proliferation
3 Enhances neutrophil, monocyte and eosinophil counts
4 Used to treat life-threatening neutropenia
5 *Side-effects:*
   (a) pericardial effusion and pericarditis
   (b) fluid retention
   (c) peritonitis
   (d) serum enzyme rises
   (e) GI disturbances.

Leukotriene antagonists (montelukast, zafirlukast)

1 Block the effects of cysteinyl leukotrienes via the cysteinyl leukotriene-1 receptor
2 Add-on therapy for mild to moderate asthma
3 Beneficial in exercise-induced asthma
4 Should not be used for treatment of an acute attack
5 Metabolised by cytochrome P450
6 May cause or aggravate Churg–Strauss syndrome
7 *Side-effects:*
   (a) headaches
   (b) GI disturbance

(c) hypersensitivity (including angio-oedema)
(d) hepatitis.

Low molecular weight heparins (LMWH)

1 At least as effective as unfractionated heparin (UFH) in the prevention of DVT and subsequent embolism and the treatment of unstable angina and PE
2 Act by selectively inhibiting factor Xa
3 Longer duration of action than UFH
4 Monitoring not required (do not prolong APTT)
5 Cannot be effectively reversed by protamine
6 Duration of action is prolonged in renal failure
7 Safe in pregnancy
8 *Side effects:*
   (a) thrombocytopenia
   (b) bleeding
   (c) osteoporosis (less than with UFH).

Clopidogrel

1 Irreversible ADP receptor antagonist (↓ platelet aggregation)
2 Reduces the risk of MI and stroke in patients with recent MI, recent stroke, or established peripheral arterial disease (CAPRIE trial)
3 Used during angioplasty and stenting
4 *Side-effects:*
   (a) bleeding
   (b) neutropenia
   (c) rash
   (d) diarrhoea.

Bupropion (Zyban®)

1 Atypical antidepressant
2 Aid to smoking cessation
3 More effective than placebo and nicotine patches
4 Most effective when combined with nicotine patches and counselling.

Abciximab

1 Monoclonal antibody that irreversibly binds glycoprotein IIb/IIIa

receptors, preventing platelet aggregation

2 *Indications:*
  (a) prevention of ischaemic complications in patients undergoing percutaneous coronary intervention (EPIC and EPILOG trials)
  (b) patients with unstable angina not responding to medical theapy and who are scheduled for percutaneous intervention (CAPTURE trial)

3 *Adverse effects:*
  (a) bleeding
  (b) thrombocytopenia.

Sildenafil (Viagra®)

1 Phosphodiesterase inhibitor (PDE5 receptor) inhibiting the breakdown of cGMP and leading to smooth muscle relaxation
2 Used for erectile dysfunction
3 Metabolised by cytochrome P450 (significantly interacts with inhibitors)
4 Reduce dose in cirrhosis and severe renal impairment
5 Nitrates contraindicated – severe hypotension occurs if used together
6 *Adverse effects:*
  (a) hypotension
  (b) priapism
  (c) headache
  (d) cardiovascular events post intercourse (?drug, ?sexual activity).

Sumatriptan

1 5-hydroxytryptamine ($5HT_1$) receptor agonist
2 Used for acute treatment of migraine and cluster headaches (effective in 80%)
3 Maintains vasoconstriction in cranial arteries preventing the vasodilator phase (headache) of migraine
4 Available as tablets, injection and nasal spray
5 Contraindicated in hemiplegic migraine, IHD, CVA and PVD
6 *Adverse effects:*
  (a) coronary artery spasm
  (b) paraesthesiae
  (c) tightness sensation over the body
  (d) hypertension.

Donepezil

1 Reversible inhibitor of acetylcholinesterase
2 Used for mild to moderate Alzheimer's disease (MMSE > 12)
3 50% of patients show slower rate of cognitive decline
4 Patient should be assessed at three months and only continue if MMSE improves or has not deteriorated and functional ability has improved.

Thiazolidinediones (pioglitazone, rosiglitazone)

1 Insulin sensitiser (increases muscle glucose uptake), reduces peripheral insulin resistance
2 Used in type 2 diabetics
3 Used in addition to metformin or sulphonylurea
4 Hyperinsulinaemia, hyperglycaemia, hypertriglyceridaemia and HbA_{1c} levels are improved
5 Induce cytochrome P450 activity
6 *Main adverse effects:*
   (a) hepatotoxicity
   (b) weight gain.

Cyclo-oxygenase-2 (COX-2) inhibitors (celecoxib, rofecoxib)

1 Selective inhibitors of COX-2 (COX-2 is induced at sites of inflammation)
2 As effective as diclofenac
3 Risk of serious GI bleeding reduced (but not excluded)
4 Shares side-effects of other NSAIDs
5 Used for RA and OA in patients with high risk of GI bleeding
6 Should not be used in patients with cardiovascular disease – do not protect against ischaemic cardiovascular events
7 Combination with low-dose aspirin leads to loss of protection against GI bleeding.

ALTERNATIVE REMEDIES

St John's wort

1 Herbal remedy, *Hypericum perforatum*

2 Used to treat depression
3 Better than placebo and equal to conventional antidepressants for mild to moderate depression
4 Cytochrome P450 inducer – may interact with numerous drugs.

Glucosamine

1 May be effective in osteoarthritis
2 May aggravate diabetes
3 Should not be given to those allergic to shellfish.

Garlic

1 May reduce total cholesterol
2 May increase bleeding in patients on warfarin and aspirin.

POISONING

Antidotes

[See Table 7, opposite]

Paracetamol

Physiology

1 In overdose paracetamol is oxidised to N-acytyl-p-benzoquinonimine (NAPQI)
2 Glutathione required to inactivate this toxic metabolite
3 In overdose glutathione levels deplete rapidly
4 Toxic liver injury occurs from NAPQI
5 12 g or more is potentially serious
6 Patients with pre-existing liver disease, alcoholism, anorexia nervosa, or those on enzyme-inducing drugs are at higher risk as they have lower glutathione stores.

Features

1 Nausea and vomiting
2 Most asymptomatic for 24 hours
3 Lactic acidosis ($<$ 12 hours)

Table 7

Drug	Antidote
Benzodiazepines	Flumazenil
Beta-blockers	Atropine
	Glucagon (7 mg)
	Pacing
Calcium antagonists	Anticholinergics
	Calcium
Carbon monoxide	Oxygen
	Hyperbaric oxygen
Cyanide	Dicobalt edetate
	Sodium thiosulphate
	Sodium nitrite
Digoxin	Digoxin-binding antibody
Methanol	Ethanol infusion
Ethylene glycol	4-methylpyrazole
Iron	Desferrioxamine
Paraquat	Fuller's earth
	IV Vitamin E
Opiates	Naloxone
Organophosphorus insecticides	Atropine
	Pralidoxime
Paracetamol	Acetylcysteine
	Methionine
Warfarin	Vitamin K
	Fresh frozen plasma (FFP)
Lead	Dimercaptosuccinic acid (DMSA)
Arsenic, mercury	Dimercaprol
Thallium	Prussian blue

4 Liver damage not detectable until 18 hours
5 Hepatic tenderness and abdominal pain on 2nd day
6 Hepatic failure at day 3–5
7 Maximal liver damage 72–96 hours
8 Renal failure (ATN) 25%
9 Hypo/hyperglycaemia
10 Arrhythmias
11 Pancreatitis
12 Cerebral oedema
13 GI bleeding.

Important prognostic markers

1 PT > 20 seconds at 24 hours, significant liver damage
2 pH < 7.3 after 24 hours = 15% survival
3 Creatinine > 300 = 23% survival
4 PT > 180 seconds = 8% survival.

Indications for a liver transplant

1 pH < 7.3 at 36 hours
2 PT > 100 seconds
3 Creatinine > 300
4 Grade 3 encephalopathy.

Management

1 Gastric lavage up to 4 hours
2 Methionine
3 Acetylcysteine (6% incidence of rash and bronchospasm)
4 Liver transplant.

Salicylates

Features

1 Mild to moderate (salicylate levels < 700 mg/l):
   (a) deafness
   (b) tinnitus
   (c) nausea
   (d) vomiting
   (e) hyperventilation
   (f) sweating
   (g) vasodilatation
   (h) tachycardia
   (i) respiratory alkalosis
   (j) metabolic acidosis
2 Severe (> 700 mg/l):
   (a) above +
   (b) confusion
   (c) delirium
   (d) hypotension
   (e) cardiac arrest

(f) acidaemia
3 Rare complications:
  (a) non-cardiogenic pulmonary oedema
  (b) cerebral oedema
  (c) convulsions
  (d) coma
  (e) encephalopathy
  (f) renal failure
  (g) tetany
  (h) hyperpyrexia
  (i) hypoglycaemia.

Management

1 Gastric lavage
2 Activated charcoal
3 Urine alkalisation with bicarbonate (not forced alkaline diuresis as this may induce pulmonary oedema)
4 Haemodialysis
5 Supportive measures.

Tricyclic antidepressants

Features

1 Anticholinergic (dry mouth, drowsiness, sinus tachycardia, urinary retention)
2 Pyramidal signs (brisk reflexes, extensor plantars)
3 Coma
4 Convulsions
5 Respiratory depression and hypoxia
6 Hypotension
7 Prolonged QT interval and arrhythmias (aggravated by acidosis)
8 Respiratory and metabolic acidosis
9 Hypothermia
10 Skin blisters.

Management

1 Gastric lavage (useful up to 12 hours due to gastroparesis)
2 Activated charcoal

3 Arrhythmias treated with bicarbonate (i.e. treat acidosis)
4 Treat convulsions with diazepam.

Carbon monoxide

Physiology

1 Carboxyhaemoglobin formed so ↓ Hb for O_2 to bind to
2 Dissociation curve shifts to left, impairing O_2 liberation.

Acute features

1 Headache
2 Dizziness
3 Nausea and vomiting
4 ↓ Consciousness
5 Hyperventilation
6 Hypotension
7 ↑ Muscle tone and reflexes
8 Metabolic acidosis
9 Rhabdomyolysis
10 MI
11 Pulmonary oedema
12 Papilloedema
13 Cerebral oedema.

Delayed complications

1 Parkinsonism
2 Cortical blindness
3 Mutism
4 Hemiplegia
5 Peripheral neuropathy.

Management

1 High-flow oxygen
2 Dantrolene (to ↓ muscle activity)
3 Hyperbaric oxygen.

Ethylene glycol (antifreeze)

Physiology

Metabolised by alcohol dehydrogenase to glycoaldehyde (CNS symptoms), glycolate (main cause of acidosis), oxalate and lactic acid.

Features

1 Inebriation but no alcohol on breath
2 Nausea and vomiting
3 Haematemesis
4 Coma
5 Convulsions
6 Papilloedema
7 Nystagmus and ophthalmoplegia
8 Hyporeflexia
9 V, VI and VII cranial nerve palsies
10 Tachypnoea and pulmonary oedema
11 Acute tubular necrosis.

Management

1 Ethanol infusion (competitively inhibits alcohol dehydrogenase)
2 4-methylpyrazole
3 Dialysis.

Iron

Features

1 Vomiting and diarrhoea
2 Abdominal pain
3 GI bleeding
4 Drowsiness
5 Coma
6 Convulsions
7 Metabolic acidosis
8 Circulatory failure
9 Jaundice and liver failure
10 Gastric stricture/pyloric stenosis (late).

Management

1 Gastric lavage
2 Supportive measures
3 Desferrioxamine
4 Dialysis
5 Exchange transfusion.

Lead

Features

1 Lethargy
2 Abdominal pain (diffuse and colicky)
3 Vomiting
4 Encephalopathy
5 Peripheral neuropathy (motor)
6 Reversible tubular dysfunction
7 Blue discoloration of gums
8 Haemolytic anaemia.

Investigations

1 Haemolysis
2 ↑ Delta-aminolaevulinic acid
3 Basophilic stippling of RBCs.

Management

Treated with dimercaptosuccinic acid (DMSA).

Theophylline

Features

1 Nausea and vomiting
2 Abdominal pain
3 Diarrhoea
4 GI bleeding
5 Hypokalaemia (marked)
6 Hyperglycaemia
7 Respiratory alkalosis

8 Metabolic acidosis
9 Arrhythmias (All)
10 Hypotension
11 Rhabdomyolysis
12 Acute renal failure
13 Restlessness
14 Headache
15 Convulsions
16 Coma.

Management

1 Activated charcoal
2 K supplements
3 Beta-blockers for arrhythmias (not in asthma)
4 Diazepam for seizures
5 Haemoperfusion.

Paraquat

Features

1 Nausea and vomiting
2 Oral and oesophageal ulcers
3 Oliguric renal failure
4 Dyspnoea
5 ARDS
6 Pulmonary fibrosis (2nd week).

Management

1 Gastric lavage with Fuller's earth
2 Oral administration of repeat-dose activated charcoal
3 Haemoperfusion/filtration
4 Intravenous Vitamin E.

Dermatology

HAIR

Causes of diffuse non-scarring alopecia

1 Endocrine:
  (a) androgenic alopecia
  (b) hypothyroidism
  (c) hypopituitarism
2 Nutritional: iron dificiency
3 Chronic disease:
  (a) liver disease
  (b) renal disease
  (c) HIV
  (d) malignancy
4 Skin diseases:
  (a) alopecia areata
  (b) psoriasis
  (c) erythroderma
5 Other systemic factors:
  (a) pregnancy
  (b) high fever
  (c) haemorrhage
  (d) starvation
  (e) surgery
  (f) emotional stress
6 Drugs:
  (a) cytotoxics
  (b) warfarin
  (c) heparin
  (d) retinoids
  (e) OCP

(f) carbimazole
(g) phenytoin
(h) carbamazepine
(i) valproate
(j) lithium
(k) allopurinol
(l) beta-blockers
(m) clofibrate
(n) colchicine.

Causes of scarring alopecia

1 Infection:
   (a) tinea capitis
   (b) staphylococcal folliculitis
   (c) syphilis
   (d) lupus vulgaris (TB)
   (e) herpes simplex and herpes zoster
2 Skin diseases:
   (a) lichen planus
   (b) BCC
   (c) pemphigoid
3 Trauma:
   (a) burns
   (b) radiotherapy
4 Systemic disorders:
   (a) sarcoid
   (b) SLE
   (c) scleroderma
   (d) metastatic carcinoma.

Causes of hirsutism (see also page 115)

Excess hair occuring in androgen-dependent areas.
  1 Polycystic ovarian disease
  2 Ovarian tumours
  3 Congenital adrenal hyperplasia
  4 Adrenal tumours
  5 Cushing's syndrome
  6 Acromegaly

7 Prolactinoma
8 Androgen therapy
9 Corticosteroids
10 Phenytoin
11 Idiopathic.

Causes of hypertrichosis

Excess hair occurring in non-androgenic areas.
1 Hypothyroidism
2 Malnutrition
3 Anorexia nervosa (lanugo hair)
4 Head injuries
5 Porphyria
6 Underlying malignancy
7 Drugs:
   (a) ciclosporin
   (b) corticosteroids
   (c) minoxidil
   (d) diazoxide
   (e) penicillamine.

NAILS

Causes of clubbing

1 Lung conditions:
   (a) carcinoma of bronchus
   (b) chronic suppurative lung disease:
       (i) bronchiectasis
       (ii) lung abscess
       (iii) empyema
       (iv) cystic fibrosis
   (c) TB
   (d) mesothelioma
   (e) CFA (cryptogenic fibrosing alveolitis)
   (f) asbestosis
2 Heart conditions:
   (a) congenital heart disease (cyanotic)

    (b) bacterial endocarditis
    (c) atrial myxoma
3 GI disease:
    (a) Crohn's/ulcerative colitis
    (b) cirrhosis
    (c) tropical sprue
    (d) malabsorption
4 Thyroid-related: acropachy
5 Familial.

Causes of nail changes

[See Table 8, opposite]

PIGMENTATION

Causes of hyperpigmentation

1 Endocrine:
    (a) Addison's disease
    (b) Cushing's syndrome
    (c) acromegaly
    (d) Nelson's syndrome
    (e) pregnancy
2 Metabolic:
    (a) porphyria
    (b) renal failure
    (c) cirrhosis
    (d) haemochromatosis
3 Nutritional:
    (a) vitamin B_{12} deficiency
    (b) pellegra
4 Other causes:
    (a) amyloid
    (b) acanthosis nigricans
    (c) lymphoma
    (d) Peutz–Jeghers' syndrome
5 Drugs:
    (a) amiodarone
    (b) OCP
    (c) minocycline.

Table 8

Nail change	Causes
Pitting	Psoriasis
	Eczema
	Alopecia areata
	Lichen planus
Ridges	Psoriasis
Dystrophy	Psoriasis
	Raynaud's
	Arterial disease
	Lichen planus
	Onychomycosis (fungal nail infection)
White spots	Trauma
Black spots	Trauma
	Naevi
	Melanoma
Red spot	Glomus tumour
Onycholysis	Psoriasis
	Onychomycosis
	Hypothyroidism
	Hyperthyroidism
	Trauma
Grooves	Acute illness (Beau's lines)
	Psoriasis
White bands	Arsenic poisoning
	Hypoalbuminaemia
Leuconychia	Cirrhosis
	Diabetes mellitus
	CCF
	Anaemia
Yellow nails	Yellow nail syndrome
Blue nails	Wilson's disease
	Melanoma
	Subungual haematoma
Koilonychia	Iron deficiency anaemia
Splinter haemorrhages	Trauma
	Bacterial endocarditis
	CTDs (connective tissue disorders)
Nail fold telangiectasia	CTDs

Causes of hypopigmentation

Localised hypopigmentation

1 Vitiligo
2 Pityriasis versicolor
3 Postinflammatory
4 Tuberous sclerosis
5 Leprosy.

Generalised hypopigmentation

1 Albinism
2 Phenylketonuria
3 Hypopituitarism.

Disorders associated with vitiligo

1 Alopecia areata
2 Halo naevus
3 Malignant melanoma
4 Thyroid disease
5 Pernicious anaemia
6 Addison's disease
7 Diabetes mellitus
8 Myasthenia gravis.

REACTION PATTERNS

Causes of orogenital ulceration

1 Behçet's disease
2 Crohn's disease
3 Ulcerative colitis
4 HCV (hepatitis C virus)
5 Reiter's disease
6 Lichen planus
7 Syphilis
8 Gonococcal infection
9 HIV

10 Pemphigus
11 Pemphigoid
12 Stevens–Johnson syndrome.

Common causes of urticaria and angio-oedema

1 Drugs:
  (a) penicillins
  (b) cephalosporins
  (c) ACE inhibitors
  (d) NSAIDs
  (e) opiates
  (f) X-ray contrast media
  (g) blood products
2 Foods:
  (a) azo dyes
  (b) benzoate preservatives
3 Arthropod reactions
4 Physical stimuli:
  (a) light pressure (dermographism)
  (b) cold
  (c) increase in body temperature (cholinergic)
  (d) light
5 Plants
6 Systemic diseases:
  (a) viral infections (hepatitis B)
  (b) SLE
  (c) vasculitides
7 Animal saliva (in atopics)
8 Inhalants:
  (a) grass pollens
  (b) house dust
9 C1 esterase inhibitor deficiency (hereditary angio-oedema).

Causes of erythroderma

Generalised exfoliative dermatitis involving > 90% of the skin.
  1 Eczema (40%)
  2 Psoriasis (25%)
  3 Mycosis fungoides (15%)

   4 Reactions to sunlight
   5 Toxic erythroderma
   6 Toxic shock syndrome
   7 Scalded skin syndrome
   8 Toxic epidermal necrolysis
   9 Infestations
10 Congenital
11 Drugs (10%):
    (a) sulphonamides
    (b) phenytoin
    (c) carbamazepine
    (d) isoniazid
    (e) lithium
    (f) captopril
    (g) allopurinol
    (h) gold
    (i) chloroquine
    (j) methyldopa.

Causes of livedo reticularis

   1 Idiopathic
   2 Physiological
   3 Vasculitis
   4 Hyperviscosity
   5 Thrombocythaemia
   6 Cryoglobulinaemia
   7 Heart failure
   8 Cholesterol emboli
   9 Paralysis
10 Drugs (amantadine).

Causes of pyoderma gangrenosum

1 Idiopathic (50%)
2 Ulcerative colitis
3 Crohn's disease
4 Rheumatoid arthritis
5 Wegener's granulomatosis
6 Myeloma

7 Paraproteinaemia
8 Leukaemia.

Causes of erythema nodosum

Systemic diseases

1 Sarcoidosis
2 Ulcerative colitis
3 Crohn's disease
4 Leukaemia
5 Hodgkin's disease
6 Behçet's disease.

Infections

1 Streptococcal infection
2 TB
3 Leprosy
4 EBV
5 Histoplasmosis
6 *Yersinia*
7 Lymphogranuloma venereum
8 Cat scratch disease
9 Tularaemia
10 Blastomycosis
11 Coccidioidomycosis.

Drugs

1 Sulphonamides
2 OCP
3 Penicillins
4 Tetracyclines
5 Sulphonylureas.

Causes of erythema multiforme

(Stevens–Johnson syndrome is a severe systemic form.)
1 Idiopathic (50%)
2 Infections:
   (a) HSV

  (b) EBV
  (c) *Mycoplasma*
  (d) *Streptococcus*
  (e) histoplasmosis
  (f) typhoid
3 SLE
4 PAN
5 Ulcerative colitis
6 Carcinoma
7 Lymphoma
8 Sarcoidosis
9 Pregnancy
10 Drugs:
  (a) penicillins
  (b) sulphonamides
  (c) co-trimoxazole
  (d) phenytoin
  (e) salicylates
  (f) barbiturates
  (g) carbamazepine
  (h) rifampicin
  (i) sulphonylureas
  (j) gold.

Causes of the Koebner phenomenon

Develops at the site of trauma.
1 Psoriasis
2 Lichen planus
3 Vitiligo
4 Viral warts
5 Molluscum contagiosum
6 Bullous pemphigoid.

SKIN MANIFESTATIONS OF SYSTEMIC DISEASE

Causes of leg ulceration

1 Trauma

2 Infections
3 Venous insufficiency
4 Peripheral vascular disease
5 Diabetes mellitus
6 Neuropathy
7 Pressure sores
8 Neoplasia
9 Pyoderma gangrenosum
10 Necrobiosis lipoidica
11 Vasculitis
12 Cholesterol emboli
13 Bullous disorders
14 TB
15 Leishmaniasis
16 Tropical ulcer
17 Haemoglobinopathy
18 Protein C/S deficiency
19 Renal failure.

Associations with internal malignancy

1 Pruritus
2 Pigmentation
3 Ichthyosis (lymphoma)
4 Acanthosis nigricans (AN) – usually gastric adenocarcinoma. Other
   associations of AN include:
   (a) obesity
   (b) inherited form
   (c) diabetes mellitus
   (d) lipodystrophy
   (e) Cushing's syndrome
   (f) acromegaly
   (g) PCOS (polycystic ovarian syndrome)
   (h) hypothyroidism
5 Acanthosis palmaris (bronchial carcinoma)
6 Erythema gyratum repens (bronchial carcinoma)
7 Acquired hypertrichosis (Hodgkin's)
8 Superficial migratory thrombophlebitis (carcinoma pancreas)
9 Necrolytic migratory erythema (glucagonoma)
10 Dermatomyositis (bronchial, breast and ovarian carcinomas)

11 Bullous pyoderma gangrenosum (leukaemia, lymphoma)
12 Pemphigoid
13 Tylosis (familial plantar and palmar keratosis associated with oesophageal carcinoma).

Skin changes in diabetes mellitus

1 Cutaneous infections
2 Neuropathic ulcers
3 Necrobiosis lipoidica
4 Diabetic dermopathy
5 Disseminated granuloma annulare
6 Bullosis diabeticorum
7 Acanthosis nigricans
8 Xanthomas and xanthelasma
9 Lipoatrophy (porcine insulins)
10 Lipohypertrophy (highly purified human insulins)
11 Scleroderma
12 Vitiligo.

Skin features of sarcoidosis

1 Erythema nodosum
2 Lupus pernio
3 Scar sarcoid
4 Plaques and subcutaneous nodules
5 Scarring alopecia.

Cutaneous manifestations of HIV and AIDS

Infections

1 Tinea and onychomycosis
2 Candidiasis
3 Hairy leucoplakia
4 Syphilis
5 Bacterial folliculitis
6 Condylomata acuminata (viral warts)
7 Molluscum contagiosum
8 Cutaneous mycobacterial infection
9 HSV

10 VZV
11 Severe aphthous stomatitis.

Inflammatory dermatoses

1 Seroconversion toxic erythema
2 Psoriasis
3 Seborrhoeic dermatitis
4 Severe drug reactions
5 Eosinophilic pustular folliculitis
6 Generalised granuloma annulare
7 Papular eruption of HIV.

Neoplasia

1 Kaposi's sarcoma
2 Cutaneous lymphoma
3 Melanoma and non-melanoma skin cancer.

Other skin manifestations

1 Acquired ichthyosis and keratoderma
2 Cutaneous and nail pigmentation.

Causes of generalised pruritus (without diagnostic skin lesions)

Endocrine

1 Hypothyroidism
2 Hyperthyroidism
3 Diabetes mellitus
4 Diabetes insipidus.

Haematological

1 Iron deficiency
2 Polycythaemia rubra vera
3 Lymphoma
4 Leukaemia
5 Myeloma.

Drugs

1 Opiates
2 Gold
3 Alcohol
4 Hepatotoxic drugs
5 OCP.

Other causes

1 Intestinal parasites
2 Scabies
3 Chronic renal failure
4 Obstructive biliary disease
5 Pregnancy
6 Psychogenic
7 Senile pruritus.

CUTANEOUS FEATURES OF SOME CONGENITAL DISORDERS

[See Table 9, opposite]

DRUGS AND THE SKIN

Causes of fixed drug eruptions

1 Phenytoin
2 Sulphonamides
3 Barbiturates
4 Dapsone
5 Quinine
6 NSAIDs
7 Tetracyclines.

Drugs that cause photosensitivity

1 Thiazides
2 Furosemide (frusemide)

Table 9

Syndrome	Skin features	Other manifestations
Xeroderma pigmentosa (AR) Defect in DNA repair	Photosensitivity, pigment changes, keratoses, skin cancers	
Tuberous sclerosis (AD)	Angiofibromas, periungual fibromas, shagreen patches, ash-leaf patches	Epilepsy, mental retardation
Neurofibromatosis (AD)	Café-au-lait spots, axillary freckling, neurofibromas	Acoustic neuromas, sarcoma, retinal Lisch nodules, epilepsy
Hereditary haemorrhagic telangiectasia (AD)	Facial and mucosal telangiectasia	Epistaxis, GI bleeding
Pseudoxanthoma elasticum (AD + AR) Defective elastin	'Chicken skin' appearance	Angioid retinal streaks, MVP, IHD, cerebral haemorrhage, GI bleeding
Peutz–Jeghers syndrome (AD)	Perioral hyperpigmentation	Multiple GI polyps, intussusception, GI malignancy
Ehlers–Danlos syndrome (AD + AR) Defective collagen	Skin fragility, tissue-paper scars, hyperelasticity	Bruising, hyperextensible joints
Cutis laxa	Lax pendulous skin, premature ageing	
Sturge–Weber syndrome	Facial port-wine stain	Epilepsy, cortical haemangioma, cortical calcification, glaucoma

DERMATOLOGY

3 ACE inhibitors
4 NSAIDs
5 Nalidixic acid
6 Tetracyclines
7 Ciprofloxacin
8 Isoniazid
9 Sulphonamides
10 Griseofulvin
11 Amiodarone
12 Sulphonylureas
13 Phenothiazines (chlorpromazine etc.)
14 Chlordiazepoxide
15 Chloroquine.

Drugs that cause a vasculitic rash

1 Allopurinol
2 Thiazides
3 Phenytoin
4 NSAIDs
5 Sulphonamides
6 Hydralazine
7 Quinidine
8 Captopril.

Drugs that cause a lichen planus-like eruption

1 Gold
2 Penicillamine
3 Streptomycin
4 Tetracycline
5 Chloroquine
6 Quinine
7 Isoniazid
8 Ethambutol
9 Thiazides
10 Furosemide (frusemide)
11 Captopril
12 Sulphonylureas
13 Phenothiazines.

DERMATITIS

Common causes of contact dermatitis

Patch testing useful for diagnosis.
1 Nickel (jewellery)
2 Cobalt
3 Chromate (leather, engineering processes)
4 Epoxy resin (glue)
5 Paraphenylenediamine (hair dyes)
6 Rubber antioxidants (gloves and shoes)
7 Preservatives
8 Lanolin (cosmetics)
9 Perfumes
10 Plants (primula, poison ivy)
11 Topical drugs:
    (a) neomycin
    (b) antihistamines
    (c) sulphonamides
    (d) local anaesthetics
12 Sticking plasters.

Aetiological factors in atopic dermatitis (eczema)

1 Atopy
2 Skin irritants
3 Contact allergens
4 Friction
5 UV light
6 Low humidity
7 Infections
8 Drugs and foods
9 Venous stasis
10 Ichthyosis.

PSORIASIS

Essential features of psoriasis

1 Associated with HLA-Cw6 (and with HLA-B27 in patients with joint disease)

2 35% have a family history
3 More common in smokers and heavy alcohol drinkers
4 Scaly, erythematous plaques affecting any part of the skin
5 Epidermal cell hyperplasia
6 Epidermal turnover time reduced from 28 days to 4 days
7 Aetiology unknown
8 Exhibits Koebner phenomenon (develops at sites of trauma)
9 Arthropathy seen in 8–10% of patients (see also page 398)
10 *Variant forms:*
   (a) chronic plaque
   (b) guttate
   (c) palmoplantar pustular
   (d) generalised pustular
   (e) erythrodermic
   (f) flexural and genital
   (g) scalp
   (h) facial
   (i) nail involvement (pitting, ridging, onycholysis, dystrophy, subungual keratosis).

Treatments for psoriasis

1 *Topical:*
   (a) tar
   (b) dithranol
   (c) steroids
   (d) calcipotriol (vitamin D analogue)
   (e) UVB
2 *Systemic:*
   (a) PUVA (psoralens and UVA) therapy
   (b) methotrexate
   (c) acitretin (retinoid)
   (d) ciclosporin
   (e) hydroxyurea
   (f) sulfasalazine.

BLISTERING SKIN DISORDERS

Causes of blistering

1 Genetic: epidermolysis bullosa

2 Physical:
   (a) heat and cold
   (b) irradiation (sun)
   (c) contact with irritants
   (d) friction
   (e) oedema
3 Inflammatory:
   (a) infections:
      (i) staphylococcal – bullous impetigo, scalded skin syndrome
      (ii) streptococcal, including necrotising fasciitis
      (iii) HSV
      (iv) herpes zoster
      (v) hand, foot and mouth disease (coxsackievirus)
      (vi) fungal
   (b) eczema
   (c) erythema multiforme
   (d) insect bites
4 Invasion:
   (a) carcinoma
   (b) amyloidosis
5 Immunological:
   (a) bullous pemphigoid
   (b) pemphigus
   (c) dermatitis herpetiformis
   (d) pemphigoid gestationis
   (e) linear IgA disease
   (f) epidermolysis bullosa
   (g) SLE
   (h) lichen planus
   (i) porphyria cutanea tarda
6 Drug reactions.

Pemphigoid

1 Autoimmune disorder of the elderly
2 Lesions are large tense blisters (up to 3 cm) with an erythematous base (subepidermal)
3 Usually on limbs, trunk and mucous membranes
4 Specific antibody (IgG) to the basement membrane of the epidermis in 70%
5 Associated with malignancy

6 Treat with high-dose prednisolone (60–80 mg/day)
7 Complete remission in one year common.

Pemphigus

1 Autoimmune blistering condition of the epidermis
2 Associated with HLA-A10, HLA-DR4
3 IgG autoantibodies to intracellular material of the epidermis in 90% (cf. pemphigoid – Ab to basement membrane)
4 Penicillamine can cause pemphigus
5 Very fragile blisters which rupture easily ('pemphig**us** lesions b**us**t')
6 Any site may be affected and blistering is usually widespread
7 Mucous membranes often involved – lesions are painful
8 Treatment with prednisolone (80–100 mg/day)
9 Azathioprine, methotrexate, ciclosporin and intravenous immunoglobulin are also used
10 Disease persists for life
11 Mortality 15–20%.

Dermatitis herpetiformis

1 Intense pruritic vesicular rash on the buttocks and extensor aspect of the elbows and knees
2 Associated with coeliac disease, HLA-B8, HLA-DR3 and HLA-DQ2
3 IgA deposited in the basement membrane zone
4 Treated with dapsone
5 Gluten-free diet results in slow improvement in rash (1–2 years)
6 Increased risk of lymphoma (reduced by gluten-free diet).

CAUSES OF SKIN TUMOURS

1 UV light
2 Thermal injury
3 X radiation
4 Hydrocarbons
5 Arsenic
6 Immunosuppression (renal transplantation)
7 Human papilloma virus (HPV)

8 Human T-cell lymphotropic virus-I (HTLV-I)
9 Human herpesvirus-8 (HHV-8) – Kaposi's sarcoma
10 Genetic predisposition (xeroderma pigmentosum)
11 Longstanding skin disease (chronic leg ulcers).

Endocrinology

THYROID HORMONES

TRH = thyrotrophin-releasing hormone
TSH = thyroid-stimulating hormone
T_4/T_3 = thyroxine/tri-iodothyronine.

Table 10

	TRH	TSH	T_4/T_3
Structure	Peptide	Peptide	Amine (acts like steroid)
Source	Hypothalamus	Anterior pituitary (basophils)	Thyroid
Acts via	Intracellular calcium	cAMP	Nuclear binding
Pregnancy	↑	↑	↑
Illness		↓	↓

Thyroid hormones are bound to thyroid-binding globulin (TBG) and thyroid-binding prealbumin (TBPA). Monoiodinase converts T_4 to T_3.

Causes of ↑ TBG and thus ↑ total T_4

1 Oestrogens
2 Chronic liver disease
3 Acute intermittent porphyria
4 Pregnancy.

Causes of ↓ TBG and thus ↓ total T_4

1 Acromegaly
2 Protein loss (malabsoption and nephrotic syndrome)
3 Androgens and steroids.

Drugs displacing T_4/T_3 from TBG

1 Aspirin
2 Phenytoin
3 Furosemide (frusemide).

Hyperthyroidism

Causes

1 Hyperthyroidism associated with overactive gland (increased uptake of radioiodine tracer):
   (a) Graves'
   (b) hot nodule
   (c) toxic multinodular goitre
2 Hyperthyroidism with normal gland (decreased/absent uptake of radioiodine tracer):
   (a) de Quervain's thyroiditis
   (b) postpartum thyroiditis
   (c) ectopic thyroid
   (d) thyroxine overdose.

Hypothyroidism

Causes

1 autoimmune:
   (a) antimicrosomal antibodies in 90%
   (b) antithyroglobulin antibodies in 60%
2 Drugs:
   (a) carbimazole
   (b) propylthiouracil
   (c) lithium
   (d) radioactive iodine
   (e) amiodarone
3 Dietary iodine deficiency.

Clinical features of thyroid disease

Table 11

Hyperthyroidism	Hypothyroidism
Weight loss (or gain)	Weight gain
Hair loss	Hair loss
Amenorrhoea	Menorrhagia
Diarrhoea	Constipation
Microcytic anaemia	Macrocytic anaemia
Leucopenia	
Proximal myopathy	Myotonia
Intermittent periodic paralysis	Cerebellar degeneration
Atrial fibrillation	Ischaemic heart disease
Cardiac failure	
Shortness of breath	Effusions

Eye signs of hyperthyroidism (see also page 341)

Table 12

	Graves'	Non-Graves'
Lid lag	✓	✓
Lid retraction	✓	✓
Periorbital oedema	✓	✗
Proptosis and exophthalmos	✓	✗
Diplopia	✓	✗
Optic nerve compression	✓	✗

Thyroid carcinoma

1 Hardly ever causes hyperthyroidism
2 10% nodules malignant
3 Types:
    (a) papillary – commonest, least aggressive
    (b) follicular – rarer, moderately aggressive
    (c) anaplastic – rarest, most aggressive
    (d) medullary – arises from C cells
    (e) lymphoma – in Hashimoto's disease.

CORTISOL

CRH = corticotrophin-releasing hormone
ACTH = adrenocorticotrophic hormone.

Table 13

	CRH	ACTH	Cortisol
Structure	Peptide	Peptide	Steroid
Source	Hypothalamus	Anterior pituitary (basophils)	Adrenal zona fasciculata
Acts via	cAMP	cAMP	Nuclear binding

Cortisol is bound to corticosteroid-binding hormone (CBG). The 10% free in plasma is the active fraction.

Cushing's syndrome/disease

Causes

1 Pituitary tumour (Cushing's disease) – 75–80%
2 Adrenal tumour – 15%
3 Ectopic ACTH (small cell carcinoma, carcinoid) – 5–10%
4 Ectopic CRH (very unusual).

Features

1 Obesity and moon face
2 Buffalo hump
3 Hirsutism
4 Acne
5 Thin skin
6 Bruising
7 Hypertension
8 Hyperglycaemia
9 Hypokalaemia
10 Osteoporosis
11 Proximal weakness
12 Psychosis.

Investigations

1 Random cortisol
2 24-hour urinary free cortisol
3 Imaging of pituitary/adrenals
4 Suppression tests.

Dexamethasone suppression test

Normal	Full suppression
Pituitary-dependent Cushing's	Some suppression
Ectopic ACTH/adrenal tumour	No suppression

Hypoadrenalism

Causes

1 Autoimmune – Addison's
2 TB
3 Metastasis
4 HIV
5 Haemorrhage (Friderichsen–Waterhouse syndrome, secondary to meningococcus)
6 Virilising hyperplasia (CAH)
7 Metyrapone
8 Pituitary failure
9 Withdrawal of longterm steroids.

Features

1 Pigmentation
2 Weight loss
3 Hypotension
4 Abdominal pain
5 Hypoglycaemia
6 Hyponatraemia
7 Hyperkalaemia
8 Hypercalcaemia
9 Normocytic anaemia with lymphocytosis.

Congenital adrenal hyperplasia

1 Autosomal recessive
2 90% is 21-hyroxylase deficiency
3 5% is 11-hyroxylase deficiency
4 High ACTH
5 Low mineralocorticoid and cortisol
6 All precursors driven into androgen production, causing virilisation, genital ambiguity etc.

Phaeochromocytoma

10% familial
10% bilateral
10% malignant (i.e. metastasis)
10% outside adrenals.

Features

1 Persistent or intermittent hypertension
2 Tachycardia and palpitations
3 Bradycardia
4 Postural hypotension
5 Pallor or flushing
6 Hyperglycaemia and glycosuria
7 Weight loss
8 Change in bowel habit
9 Raynaud's phenomenon.

Investigations

1 Urinary metanephrins
2 CT scan
3 MRI (T_2-weighted)
4 MIBG scan.

Note: invasive procedures or radiocontrast studies need α- and β-blockade to prevent hypertensive crisis.

MULTIPLE ENDOCRINE NEOPLASIA (MEN)

All forms are autosomal dominant.

MEN I (chromosome 11)

1 **P**arathyroid
2 **P**ancreas, including:
  (a) insulinoma
  (b) gastrinoma
  (c) glucagonoma
  (d) VIPoma
  (e) PPPoma
3 **P**ituitary (60% prolactinoma).

MEN IIA (chromosome 10)

1 Medullary carcinoma of thyroid (MCT)
2 Phaeochromocytoma
3 Parathyroid.

MEN IIB

1 MCT
2 Phaeochromocytoma
3 Parathyroid
4 Marfanoid
5 Mucosal neuromas.

HYPOTHALMIC AND PITUITARY HORMONES

Important anatomical associations

1 Optic chiasm (bitemporal hemianopia)
2 Cavernous sinus containing branches of cranial nerves III, IV, V (ophthalmic only) and VI
3 Sphenoidal sinus (surgery).

Pituitary tumours

1 Microadenoma < 1 cm; macroadenoma > 1 cm

2 Nearly always benign, but can get secondaries from breast carcinoma
3 50% of all tumours are non-secreting.

Prolactin

Excess secretion is the only cause of galactorrhoea. Under negative control of the hypothalamus by dopamine, i.e. **increased** dopamine results in **decreased** prolactin.

Causes of raised prolactin

1 Stress, e.g. epileptic fit
2 Pregnancy
3 Oestrogens (oral contraceptive)
4 Dopamine antagonist drugs (metoclopramide, phenothiazines)
5 PCOS
6 Damage to hypothalamus or pituitary stalk
7 Renal or hepatic failure.

Hyperprolactinaemia may cause secondary hypogonadism.

Causes of low prolactin

Dopamine and dopamine agonists (bromocriptine).

Prolactinoma

1 25% of all pituitary tumours
2 Invariably large in men, small in women
3 May be part of MEN I.

Growth hormone (GH)

1 Peptide hormone from anterior pituitary
2 Under control of growth hormone-releasing hormone (GHRH) from the hypothalamus, and somatostatin
3 Secreted in pulsatile fashion mainly at night – levels may be undetectable between pulses
4 Acts directly and via stimulation of insulin-like growth factor-1 (IGF-1) produced in the liver.

Causes of GH deficiency

1 Pituitary tumours
2 Parapituitary tumour (craniopharyngioma)
3 Trauma (surgery)
4 Infarction (pituitary apoplexy – bleed into the tumour)
5 Pituitary infection (abscess, TB).

Features of GH deficiency

1 Decreased energy and exercise tolerance
2 Decreased bone density
3 Reduced muscle mass
4 Increased body fat
5 Increased lipids
6 Reduced cardiac output.

Acromegaly

1 Usually due to pituitary tumour
2 12% of all pituitary tumours secrete GH. Of these, 90% are macroadenomas
3 Rarely due to ectopic GHRH from carcinoid
4 Diagnosis by failure of GH to suppress to oral glucose load – may get a paradoxical rise.

Features

1 Coarse facial appearance
2 Large hands/feet
3 Enlarged lower jaw
4 Hypertension
5 Diabetes mellitus
6 Increased cardiovascular mortality
7 Obstructive sleep apnoea
8 Carpal tunnel syndrome
9 Hyperhydrosis
10 Arthropathy
11 Renal stones
12 Increased colonic malignancy
13 LVH and cardiomyopathy.

Treatment

1 Pituitary surgery
2 Octreotide (somatostatin analogue)
3 Pituitary irradiation
4 Bromocriptine.

Vasopressin

Peptide hormone, secreted by the hypothalamus and stored in the posterior pituitary.

Cranial diabetes insipidus

Caused by damage to hypothalamic nuclei by:
1 Pituitary tumours
2 Parapituitary tumour (craniopharyngioma)
3 Trauma and surgery
4 Infiltration of hypothalamus by sarcoid, histiocytosis X
5 Idiopathic.

SEX HORMONES

LH = luteinising hormone
FSH = follicle-stimulating hormone
Glycoproteins – α and β subunits.

Precocious puberty

Gonadotrophin-dependent (true) causes

1 Idiopathic
2 CNS/hypothalamic disease (tumour, trauma, infection).

Gonadotrophin-independent causes

1 CAH
2 Excess testosterone
3 Adrenal or ovarian tumour
4 Oestrogen therapy
5 Severe hypothyroidism.

Delayed puberty

1 Overt or occult systemic disease
2 Anorexia
3 Genetic disorders, e.g. Turner's, Klinefelter's, Noonan's, androgen insensitivity.

Hypogonadism in males

Causes

1 Hypopituitarism
2 Selective gonadal deficiency
3 Hyperprolactinaemia
4 Primary congenital gonadal disease (Klinefelter's, anorchia)
5 Primary acquired gonadal disease:
    (a) torsion, castration, radiotherapy
    (b) renal failure, liver failure
6 Androgen receptor deficiency.

Features

1 Loss of libido
2 Increasing pitch of voice
3 Loss of male pattern of hair distribution
4 Decreased testicular size
5 Loss of erectile and ejaculatory function
6 Failure of spermatogenesis
7 Loss of muscle bulk.

Hypogonadism in females

Causes

1 Ovarian failure (total):
    (a) dysgenesis
    (b) steroid biosynthetic defect
    (c) oophorectomy
    (d) radio/chemotherapy
2 Ovarian failure (partial):
    (a) polycystic ovary syndrome

    (b) resistant ovary syndrome
3 Gonadotrophin failure:
    (a) hypothalamo-pituitary disease
    (b) Kallmann's syndrome
    (c) anorexia
    (d) systemic illness
    (e) hypothyroidism.

Features

1 Thinning and loss of pubic hair
2 Small atrophic breasts
3 Vaginal dryness and dyspareunia
4 Atrophy of vulva and vagina
5 Osteoporosis
6 Infertility
7 Amenorrhoea.

Causes of gynaecomastia

Physiological

1 Neonate
2 Puberty
3 Old age.

Pathological

1 Hyper/hypothyroidism
2 Chronic liver disease
3 Tumours producing oestrogen (adrenal, testicular)
4 Tumours producing HCG (lung, testis)
5 Acromegaly
6 Carcinoma of breast
7 Leprosy
8 Starvation.

Drugs (see also page 58)

1 Oestrogens
2 Digoxin

3 Spironolactone
4 Cimetidine
5 Cyproterone
6 Gonadotrophins
7 Cannabis.

Causes of hirsutism (see also page 82)

With virilisation

1 Severe polycystic ovarian syndrome
2 Ovarian neoplasm
3 Adrenal tumour
4 Congenital adrenal hyperplasia.

Without virilisation

1 Familial
2 Idiopathic
3 Mild polycystic ovarian syndrome
4 Late-onset CAH.

Drugs

1 Androgens
2 Phenytoin
3 Some progesterogens.

INSULIN

1 Peptide hormone
2 Synthesised as proinsulin
3 Cleaved to form insulin and C-peptide on secretion
4 Short plasma half-life
5 Acts via receptor tyrosine kinases
6 Stimulates hepatic glycogen and fat synthesis
7 Stimulates muscle to synthesise glycogen and protein

8 Stimulates adipose tissue to synthesise triglycerides
9 Stimulates uptake of glucose and amino acids by muscle
10 Stimulates cellular uptake of potassium.

WHO definition of diabetes

All definitions are based on venous plasma values of glucose during oral glucose tolerance test.

Table 14

	Plasma glucose (mmol/l)	
	Fasting	2 hours post-glucose load
Diabetes mellitus	≥ 7.0	≥ 11.1
Impaired glucose tolerance	< 7.0	7.8–11.0
Normal	< 7.0	< 7.8

OR
Single fasting glucose ≥ 7.0 mmol/l and characteristic diabetic symptoms.
OR
Fasting glucose of ≥ 7.0 mmol/l on two separate occasions without characteristic symptoms.

Types of diabetes and their aetiology

Type 1 diabetes mellitus

1 10% of cases
2 Juvenile onset
3 Insulin-dependent
4 Antibodies to islet cells in pancreas cause autoimmune destruction of insulin-producing cells
5 60–90% have islet-cell antibodies at diagnosis
6 50% concordance in identical twins
7 10–20% risk to child if both parents have the condition
8 HLA-DR3/4 associated in 95%
9 HLA-DR2 protective
10 Commonest in Caucasians.

Type 2 diabetes mellitus

1 85% of cases
2 Maturity onset
3 Non-insulin-dependent
4 Peripheral cell resistance to insulin
5 No associated autoantibodies
6 Identical twins – near 100% incidence
7 70–100% risk if both parents have the condition
8 No HLA association
9 Commonest in Afro-Caribbeans and South Asians.

Secondary diabetes (5%)

1 Due to pancreatic disorders causing insulin deficiency:
  (a) pancreatitis
  (b) carcinoma of the pancreas
  (c) cystic fibrosis
  (d) haemochromatosis
  (e) pancreatectomy
2 Due to insulin resistance:
  (a) endocrine causes:
    (i) Cushing's syndrome
    (ii) thyrotoxicosis
    (iii) acromegaly
    (iv) phaeochromocytoma
    (v) polycystic ovarian syndrome
    (vi) glucagonoma
  (b) drugs:
    (i) steroids
    (ii) thiazides
  (c) genetic causes:
    (i) congenital lipodystrophy
    (ii) Friedreich's ataxia.

Oral hypoglycaemic agents

Biguanides (metformin)

1 Reduce glucose absorption from gut; increase insulin sensitivity
2 Duration of action 12–20 hours

3 Excreted unchanged in urine
4 Side-effects – anorexia, diarrhoea, epigastric pain
5 Contraindicated in renal/hepatic failure, may cause lactic acidosis.

Alpha-glucosidase inhibitors (acarbose)

1 Slow carbohydrate absorption
2 Not complicated by hypoglycaemia.

Sulphonylureas

1 Increase insulin secretion, both basal and stimulated
2 Reduce peripheral resistance to insulin
3 Albumin-bound, so may be displaced by other drugs
4 Effects may be reduced by steroids or thiazide diuretic therapy.

Table 15

Suphonylurea	Duration of action (hours)	Excretion/metabolism	Side-effects
Tolbutamide	6–8	Hepatic	Hypoglycaemia – may be prolonged in drugs with long half-life; skin rashes
Gliclazide	10–12	Hepatic and renal	
Glibenclamide	12–20	Hepatic and renal	
Chlorpropamide	36–48	Renal	Hypoglycaemia; facial flushing with alcohol; cholestatic jaundice; SIADH

Diabetic emergencies

Diabetic ketoacidosis (DKA)

1 Usually type 1 DM, may be first presentation
2 State of uncontrolled catabolism due to insulin deficiency
3 Usually precipitated by insulin omission or intercurrent illness
4 Vomiting, dehydration, thirst, abdominal pain, hyperventilation, decreased conscious level
5 Ketonuria, hyperglycaemia, metabolic acidosis, hyperkalaemia, may be renal failure

6 Treat with rehydration, sliding-scale insulin, and consider antibiotics and low molecular weight heparin.

Hyperosmolar non-ketotic state (HONK)

1 Usually type 2 DM
2 Insidious onset
3 May be due to glucose overload or steroid/thiazide treatment in undiagnosed diabetic
4 Profound dehydration and hyperglycaemia
5 Vomiting, acidosis and hyperkalaemia infrequent
6 Raised osmolality
7 Treatment with rehydration; may show dramatic glucose fall with only a small amount of insulin.

Hypoglycaemia

Causes in diabetes

1 Excess insulin/sulphonylurea treatment
2 Inadequate carbohydrate intake.

Causes unrelated to diabetes

1 Insulinoma
2 Malignancy (due to IGF-2)
3 Adrenal failure
4 Pituitary failure
5 Hepatic failure
6 End-stage renal failure (ESRF)
7 Chronic alcohol abuse
8 Sepsis
9 Inherited metabolic disorder
10 Post-gastrectomy.

Complications of diabetes

Macrovascular

1 Increasing risk of cerebrovascular disease, ischaemic heart disease and myocardial infarction, and peripheral vascular disease
2 Independent of glycaemic control and HbA_{1c} (glycosylated haemoglobin)

3 Multifactorial: increased age, duration of diabetes, systolic hypertension, hyperlipidaemia and proteinuria all important. Proteinuria is a strong risk factor for IHD.

Microvascular

Progress of microvascular change is dependent on the degree of glycaemic control.

Retinopathy (see also page 339)

1 Affects 90% at some time
2 Commonest cause of blindness in under-60s
3 Background (early) vs. proliferative (late)
4 After 20 years, proliferative retinopathy in 60% of type 1 DM and 20% of type 2 DM.

Neuropathy

1 Affects 70–90% at some time
2 Huge range of presentations and severity
3 May be due to ischaemia in vasa nervorum.

Autonomic neuropathy

1 General and gustatory sweating
2 Postural hypotension
3 Gastroparesis
4 Diarrhoea
5 Cardiac arrhythmias.

Nephropathy (see also page 294)

1 Affects 30–40% at some time
2 Commonest cause of death in young diabetics
3 Microalbuminuria = 25–250 mg/day
4 Macroalbuminuria > 250 mg/day
5 With persistent proteinuria, progression to ESRF is likely in 8–10 years
6 ACE inhibitors beneficial.

Pregnancy and diabetes

Poorly controlled diabetes in the mother is associated with:
1 Fetal macrosomia
2 Intrauterine death
3 Hydramnios
4 Pre-eclampsia
5 Hyaline membrane disease in the newborn
6 Neonatal hypoglycaemia.

DKA carries 50% mortality. Close monitoring important.

Gestational diabetes

1 Glucose intolerance during pregnancy which remits after delivery
2 Usually asymptomatic
3 Treatment with diet, but most will need insulin (oral agents may harm fetus)
4 Likely to recur in subsequent pregnancies
5 Increased incidence of type 2 DM later.

Gastroenterology

GI PHYSIOLOGY

Gut Hormones

[See Table 16, overleaf]

Control of gastric acid secretion

Stimulators of acid secretion

1 Vagus:
   (a) direct – stimulates acetylcholine receptors on the parietal cell
   (b) indirect – increases gastrin secretion
2 Gastrin
3 Histamine (H_2 receptors).

Inhibitors of acid secretion

1 Higher centres
2 Low pH
3 CCK
4 GIP
5 Secretin
6 Protaglandin E_2 (misoprostol)
7 H_2 receptor antagonists (ranitidine, cimetidine)
8 Proton pump inhibitors (omeprazole etc.).

THE MOUTH

Causes of mouth ulcers

Systemic diseases

1 Crohn's disease
2 Coeliac disease

Table 16

Hormone	Source	Stimulus	Action
Gastrin	G cells in antrum	Gastric distension	Secretion of pepsin, gastric acid and intrinsic factor
		Amino acids in antrum	
Cholecystokinin-pancreozymin (CCK-PZ)	Duodenum and jejunum	Fat, amino acids and peptides in the small bowel	Pancreatic secretion
			Gallbladder contraction
			Delays gastric emptying
Secretin	Duodenum and jejunum	Acid in the small bowel	Pancreatic bicarbonate secretion
			Delays gastric emptying
Motilin	Duodenum and jejunum	Acid in the small bowel	Increases motility
Vasoactive intestinal peptide (VIP)	Small intestine	Neural stimulation	Inhibits gastric acid and pepsin secretion
			Stimulates secretion by intestine and pancreas
Gastric inhibitory peptide (GIP)	Duodenum and jejunum	Glucose, fats and amino acids	Inhibits gastric acid secretion
			Stimulates insulin secretion
			Reduces motility
Somatostatin	D cells in pancreas	Vagal and beta-adrenergic stimulation	Inhibits gastric and pancreatic secretion
Pancreatic polypeptide	PP cells in pancreas	Protein-rich meal	Inhibition of pancreatic and biliary secretion

3 Glandular fever
4 Tuberculosis
5 Behçet's disease
6 Reiter's syndrome
7 Wegener's granulomatosis
8 SLE
9 Syphilis.

Dermatological conditions

1 Pemphigus vulgaris
2 Pemphigoid
3 Erythema multiforme and Stevens–Johnson syndrome
4 Lichen planus.

Local causes

1 Aphthous
2 Herpes simplex (HSV 1)
3 Coxsackie A virus
4 *Fusobacterium nucleatum*
5 *Borrelia vincenti*
6 Denture gingivitis
7 Trauma
8 Carcinoma (squamous, adenocarcinoma)
9 Idiopathic
10 Actinomycosis.

Causes of white oral plaques

1 Candidiasis
2 Squamous cell carcinoma
3 Leukoplakia
4 Hairy leukoplakia
5 Frictional keratosis
6 Condylomata latum of secondary syphilis.

Causes of pigmentation of oral mucosa

1 Addison's disease
2 Peutz–Jeghers' disease

3 Lead poisoning
4 Smoker's melanosis
5 Malignant melanoma
6 Von Recklinghausen's disease of the skin
7 Albright's syndrome
8 Acanthosis nigricans
9 Drugs:
   (a) chloroquine
   (b) minocycline
   (c) cyclophosphamide.

Causes of glossitis

1 Nutritional deficiencies:
   (a) B_{12}
   (b) iron
   (c) riboflavin
   (d) niacin
   (e) pyridoxine
2 Syphilis
3 Inhalation burns
4 Ingestion of corrosive materials.

Causes of macroglossia

1 Primary
2 Amyloidosis
3 Acromegaly
4 Hypothyroidism
5 Tongue haemangiomas
6 Neurofibromatosis.

Tongue cancer

1 Squamous cell
2 *Risk factors:*
   (a) smoking
   (b) alcohol
   (c) chilli consumption
   (d) betel nuts
   (e) HIV

(f) HPV-16 infection
3 Leukoplakia and submucosal fibrosis are precancerous lesions
4 Presents as non-resolving lump or oral ulcer
5 Metastasises to sudmandibular and upper cervical nodes
6 Treatment by excision.

Causes of bilateral parotid swelling

1 Infections:
   (a) mumps
   (b) bacterial parotitis
2 Sarcoidosis
3 Sjögren's syndrome
4 Cirrhosis
5 Alcoholism
6 Lymphoma
7 Parotid tumours
8 Cystic fibrosis
9 Diabetes
10 Amyloidosis
11 Anorexia nervosa
12 Malabsorption
13 Hyperlipidaemia
14 Acromegaly
15 Drugs:
   (a) lead
   (b) iodides
   (c) thiouracil.

Causes of xerostomia

Dryness of the mouth caused by reduced secretion of saliva.
1 Mumps
2 Dehydration
3 Sjögren's syndrome
4 Granulomatous disease (sarcoid, TB, leprosy)
5 Amyloidosis
6 HIV
7 Diabetes mellitus
8 Graft- versus-host disease

9 Depression
10 Radiotherapy
11 Drugs:
 (a) anticholinergics
 (b) neuroleptics
 (c) antihistamines
 (d) antidepressants.

UPPER GI TRACT

Causes of upper GI bleeding

Common

1 Duodenal ulcer – 35%
2 Gastric ulcer – 20%
3 Gastric erosions – 18%
4 Mallory–Weiss tear – 10%.

Uncommon (5% or less)

1 Duodenitis
2 Oesophageal varices
3 Oesophagitis
4 Upper GI neoplasia.

Rare 1% or less

1 Angiodysplasia
2 Hereditary haemorrhagic telangiectasia
3 Portal hypertensive gastropathy
4 Aorto-duodenal fistula
5 Mesenteric ischaemia
6 Munchausen's syndrome
7 Watermelon stomach.

Causes of dysphagia

1 GORD and oesophagitis
2 Stroke
3 Oesophageal cancer

4 Hiatus hernia
5 Achalasia
6 Peptic strictures
7 Oesophageal web or ring
8 Plummer–Vinson (or Paterson–Brown–Kelly) syndrome –
   oesophageal web, iron deficiency anaemia and oesophageal cancer
9 Gastric cancer
10 Pharyngeal cancer
11 Extrinsic pressure from:
   (a) lung cancers
   (b) mediastinal cancers
   (c) retrosternal goitre
   (d) enlarged left atrium
   (e) lymphadenopathy
12 Pharyngeal pouch
13 Oesophageal diverticulum
14 Oesophageal candidiasis
15 Herpes simplex oesophagitis
16 Systemic sclerosis
17 Bulbar palsy (MND)
18 Pseudobulbar palsy
19 Myasthenia gravis
20 Parkinson's disease
21 Syringomyelia
22 Chagas' disease
23 Globus hystericus
24 Diffuse oesophageal spasm
25 Nutcracker oesophagus
26 Corkscrew oesophagus.

Oesophageal cancer

1 Squamous or adenocarcinoma (arises from Barrett's epithelium)
2 Mostly middle third
3 Incidence rising
4 50% have metastases at diagnosis
5 5% five-year survival
6 *Risk factors:*
   (a) smoking
   (b) alcohol

    (c) achalasia
    (d) Barrett's oesophagus
    (e) tylosis (autosomal dominant palmar and plantar keratosis)
    (f) coeliac disease
    (g) Plummer–Vinson syndrome
    (h) bile acid reflux
7 *Symptoms:*
    (a) dysphagia for solids then liquids
    (b) weight loss
    (c) pain and dyspepsia
    (d) haematemesis and melaena
8 *Diagnosis:*
    (a) endoscopy
    (b) barium swallow
    (c) CT and laparoscopy for staging
9 *Treatment:*
    (a) surgery
    (b) endoscopy and stenting
    (c) radiotherapy
    (d) chemotherapy (cisplatin and fluorouracil).

Barrett's oesophagus

1 Complication of long-term gastro-oesophageal reflux
2 Present in 11% of patients with symptoms of GORD
3 Lower oesophageal squamous mucosa replaced by metaplastic columnar mucosa in response to acid
4 Predisposes to adenocarcinoma (30–40-fold increase in risk with >2 cm segment)
5 Patients with dysplasia on biopsy are at highest risk of developing carcinoma
6 Treatment with long-term protein pump inhibitors (PPIs), but this will not reverse it.

Hiatus hernia

1 Herniation of proximal stomach into the thoracic cavity
2 Sliding (80%) or rolling (20%)
3 Common, incidence 30% >50 years
4 50% have GORD
5 *Diagnosis* by barium meal or gastroscopy

6 *Treatment:*
   (a) weight loss
   (b) antacids
   (c) PPIs
   (d) surgery.

Gastro-oesophageal reflux disease (GORD) and oesophagitis

1 Very common
2 *Symptoms:*
   (a) chest pain – retrosternal discomfort
   (b) dysphagia
   (c) waterbrash
   (d) nocturnal cough and wheeze
   (e) belching
3 *Complications:*
   (a) oesophagitis/ulcer
   (b) stricture
   (c) iron deficiency anaemia
   (d) Barrett's oesophagus
   (e) pulmonary aspiration
4 *Aggravating factors:*
   (a) obesity
   (b) smoking
   (c) alcohol
   (d) coffee
   (e) large meals
   (f) hiatus hernia
   (g) pregnancy
   (h) systemic sclerosis
   (i) fatty foods
   (j) chocolate
   (k) drugs – nitrates, anticholinergics, NSAIDs, bisphosphonates
5 *Investigation:*
   (a) symptoms do not correlate with endoscopic appearance (but essential to exclude Barrett's)
   (b) 24-hour pH monitoring (symptoms correlate with low pH)
6 *Treatment:*
   (a) lifestyle changes
   (b) antacids

(c) H$_2$ antagonists
(d) PPIs
(e) promotility agents – metoclopramide, domperidone
(f) fundoplication (open/laparoscopic).

Achalasia

1 Lack of relaxation of the lower oesophageal sphincter, abnormal peristalsis and dilated oesophagus proximal to the sphincter
2 Loss of ganglia from the myenteric plexus
3 *Symptoms:*
   (a) dysphagia – solids and liquids from onset
   (b) regurgitation
   (c) chest pain
   (d) weight loss
   (e) aspiration pneumonia
4 *Diagnosis* by barium swallow or oesophageal manometry
5 *Complication* – squamous carcinoma
6 *Treament:*
   (a) endoscopic dilatation
   (b) surgical myotomy
   (c) botulinum toxin.

Helicobacter pylori

1 Spiral, flagellate, Gram-negative, microaerophilic bacterium
2 Cag A +ve *H. pylori* are pathogenic
3 Produces urease that forms ammonia to neutralise the surrounding area
4 More common in low socio-economic groups (and gastroenterologists!)
5 *Associated diseases:*
   (a) acute gastritis (some patients have an acute illness when infected)
   (b) chronic gastritis:
       (i) pangastritis – leads to atrophic gastritis
       (ii) antral gastritis – may lead to DU
       (iii) gastritis of corpus – may lead to GU and adenocarcinoma
   (c) DU (95% *H. pylori* +ve)
   (d) GU (80% *H. pylori* +ve)
   (e) gastric adenocarcinoma

(f)   gastric lymphoma – MALToma
(g)   ? functional dyspepsia
6   *Methods of detection:*
   (a)   rapid urease test at endoscopy (95% spec., 95% sens.)
   (b)   histology (100% spec., 85% sens.)
   (c)   culture (100% spec., 95% sens – useful for sensitivities to antibiotics)
   (d)   urea breath test (95% spec., 97% sens.)
   (e)   serology (50–90% spec., 70–90% sens.)
7   Eradicate with triple therapy, e.g. omeprazole, metronidazole and clarithromycin.

Causes of gastritis

1   *H. pylori*
2   Atrophic gastritis
3   Pernicious anaemia
4   NSAIDs
5   Alcohol
6   Stress
7   Infections in the immunocompromised:
   (a)   CMV
   (b)   herpes
   (c)   *Candida*
   (d)   TB
8   Gastric ischaemia
9   Radiation
10   Corrosive substances
11   Ménétrier's disease
12   Eosinophilic gastritis
13   Granulomatous gastritis
14   Watermelon stomach.

Risk factors for peptic ulcer disease

1   *H. Pylori*
2   High alcohol intake
3   NSAID use
4   High-dose steroids
5   Male sex

6 Smoking
7 Zollinger–Ellison syndrome
8 Stress (Curling's ulcer)
9 Head trauma (Cushing's ulcer)
10 Blood group **O** (du-**o**-denal).

Risk factors for gastric carcinoma

1 Japanese
2 *H. Pylori*
3 Pernicious anaemia
4 Chronic atrophic gastritis
5 Male sex
6 Blood group **A** (g-**a**-stric)
7 Gastric resection (increased bile reflux)
8 Nitrosamines in diet
9 Adenomatous polyps > 2 cm in stomach.

Gastrinoma

1 Leads to Zollinger–Ellison syndrome
2 Usually pancreatic (also stomach, duodenum or adjacent tissues)
3 50–60% malignant
4 10% multiple
5 Associated with MEN (30%)
6 Signs:
   (a) single ulcer (most common endoscopic finding)
   (b) multiple peptic ulcers
   (c) steatorrhoea and diarrhoea (40%)
7 *Diagnosis:*
   (a) high serum fasting gastrin with little further increase with pentagastrin
   (b) CT to find tumour (40% less than 1 cm) and assess for metastases
8 *Treatment:*
   (a) high-dose omeprazole 80–120 mg daily
   (b) surgery to resect adenoma
   (c) octreotide to reduce diarrhoea.

Causes of hypergastrinaemia

1 Achlorhydria
2 PPI therapy

3 Zollinger–Ellison syndrome
4 *H. pylori*
5 Antral G-cell hyperplasia
6 CRF
7 Gastric outlet obstruction.

Complications of gastrectomy

1 Early satiety
2 Abdominal fullness
3 Dumping syndrome (40%)
4 Postprandial hypoglycaemia
5 Bile reflux
6 Weight loss and malnutrition
7 Iron deficiency anaemia (common)
8 Malabsorption and bacterial overgrowth
9 B_{12} deficiency
10 Osteoporosis/osteomalacia
11 Gallstones
12 Anastomotic ulcers
13 May predispose to carcinoma in the gastric remnant.

Causes of vomiting

GI irritation

1 Enteritis
2 Drugs (NSAIDs, alcohol)
3 Poisons
4 Gastritis
5 Gastric ulcer.

Obstruction

1 Atresia
2 Stricture – malignant, benign
3 Stenosis
4 Intussusception
5 Volvulus
6 Hernia
7 Paralytic ileus.

Intra-abdominal inflammation

1 Hepatitis
2 Pancreatitis
3 Appendicitis
4 Pyelonephritis
5 Cholecystitis.

Metabolic and endocrine

1 Diabetic ketoacidosis/hypoglycaemia
2 Pregnancy
3 Uraemia
4 Hypoadrenalism
5 Hypercalcaemia.

Neurological

1 Psychogenic
2 Severe pain
3 Drugs (opioids, chemotherapeutic drugs)
4 Migraine
5 Motion sickness
6 Meningitis
7 Ménière's disease
8 Labyrinthitis
9 Raised ICP (benign, malignant).

Miscellaneous causes

1 Acute dilatation of the stomach
2 Cyclical vomiting
3 Radiation sickness.

SMALL BOWEL DISORDERS

Causes of malabsorption

Conditions within the gut lumen

1 Lack of pancreatic enzymes:

(a) chronic pancreatitis
(b) cystic fibrosis
(c) pancreatic carcinoma
(d) genetic pancreatic insufficiency
2 Lack of bile salts:
(a) obstructive jaundice
(b) cholestatic liver disease
(c) bile salt loss
(d) bacterial overgrowth
3 Infective:
(a) traveller's diarrhoea
(b) intestinal TB
(c) parasitic disease (especially *Giardia*, helminths)
(d) HIV
(e) tropical sprue
4 Inadequate mixing and motility disorders:
(a) post-gastrectomy
(b) thyrotoxicosis
(c) diabetes (autonomic neuropathy)
(d) systemic sclerosis.

Conditions in the gut mucosa

1 Coeliac disease
2 Disaccharidase deficiency (lactase, sucrase-isomaltase deficiency)
3 Post-infectious malabsorption
4 Whipple's disease
5 Immunodeficiency (hypogammaglobulinaemia)
6 Crohn's disease
7 Cow's milk sensitivity in infants.

Structural disorders

1 Intestinal/gastric resection
2 Radiation enteritis
3 Mesenteric arterial insufficiency
4 Small intestinal lymphoma or other malignancy
5 Amyloidosis.

Conditions outside the gut mucosa

Intestinal lymphangiectasia.

Drugs

1 Alcohol
2 Neomycin
3 Metformin
4 Cholestyramine
5 Colchicine.

Tests for malabsorption

Table 17

Test	Use
Iron/ferritin	↓ Proximal small bowel disease
Folate	↓ Proximal small bowel disease
	↑ Bacterial overgrowth
B_{12}	↓ Pernicious anaemia
	↓ Bacterial overgrowth
	↓ Terminal ileal disease
	↓ Chronic pancreatitis
	Schilling test useful to differentiate further
Faecal fat	Steatorrhoea
D-xylose test	↓ Small bowel disease
	Normal in pancreatic disease
PABA test	↓ Pancreatic disease
Pancreolauryl test	
Hydrogen breath test	↑ Bacterial overgrowth
Duodenal biopsy	Histological diagnosis, e.g. coeliac disease
Jejunal aspirate	Bacterial overgrowth
Barium follow through/small bowel enema	Structural defects in the small bowel, e.g. terminal ileal stricture, diverticulae
Se HCAT	Bile acid malabsorption

Causes of infective diarrhoea (see also page 240)

Bloody diarrhoea (enterocolitis)

1 Campylobacter spp.
2 Shigella spp.
3 Salmonella spp.
4 Clostridium difficile
5 Escherichia coli (enteroinvasive)
6 Yersinia spp.
7 Amoebiasis (Entamoeba histolytica)
8 Schistosomiasis.

Watery diarrhoea

1 Viral – rotavirus, Norwalk virus and adenovirus
2 Shigella spp.
3 Salmonella spp.
4 E. coli (enterotoxigenic)
5 Vibrio cholerae (cholera)
6 Giardiasis
7 Cryptosporidium parvum.

Causes of non-infective diarrhoea

Bowel disease

1 Diverticulosis
2 Irritable bowel syndrome
3 Disaccharidase deficiency
4 Carcinoma of bowel (presentation)
5 Villous adenoma of rectum
6 Intestinal lymphoma
7 Post-vagotomy/gastrectomy
8 Inflammatory bowel disease
9 Small bowel malabsorption
10 Bowel ischaemia
11 Bile acid malabsorption
12 Microscopic/lymphocytic/collagenous colitis.

Endocrine conditions

1 Thyrotoxicosis

2 Diabetes (autonomic neuropathy)
3 Adrenal insufficiency
4 Carcinoid syndrome
5 VIPomas
6 Gastrinomas
7 Medullary carcinoma of thyroid.

Other causes

1 Laxative abuse
2 Connective tissue disorders (scleroderma, SLE, MCTD)
3 Amyloidosis
4 AIDS
5 Allergy
6 Immunoglobulin deficiency
7 Drugs:
   (a) antibiotics
   (b) magnesium-based antacids
   (c) digoxin
   (d) NSAIDs
   (e) alcohol
   (f) chemotherapy.

Causes of bacterial overgrowth

1 ↓ Acid:
   (a) atrophic gastritis
   (b) vagotomy
   (c) PPIs and H_2 blockers
2 Blind loops
3 Diverticulae
4 Fistulae
5 Obstruction:
   (a) adhesions
   (b) strictures
6 Disordered motility:
   (a) systemic sclerosis
   (b) diabetic autonomic neuropathy
   (c) amyloid
7 Hypogammaglobulinaemia

8 Cirrhosis.

Coeliac disease

1 Sensitivity to gluten (gliaden fraction) leads to villous atrophy
2 Gluten present in bran, oats, wheat and rye
3 Found in 0.1–0.2% of population (more common in west of Ireland – 1 in 300)
4 HLA-B8 and HLA-DR3 in 90% – associated with organ-specific autoimmune diseases (DM, thyroid disease, Addison's, fibrosing alveolitis and SLE)
5 *Clinical features:*
   (a) diarrhoea
   (b) steatorrhoea (vitamin A, D, E and K deficiencies)
   (c) weight loss
   (d) growth retardation
   (e) oral aphthous ulcers
   (f) malaise
   (g) anaemia (folate, B_{12}, iron)
   (h) bruising
   (i) increased incidence of all GI malignancy (especially small bowel lymphoma)
   (j) dermatitis herpetiformis (see also page 100)
   (k) hyposplenism
   (l) osteomalacia
   (m) IgA deficiency (5%)
6 Diagnosis:
   (a) duodenal/jejunal biopsy
   (b) endomysial Ab (95% positive predictive value)
   (c) antigliadin Ab
   (d) antireticulin Ab
7 *Treatment* with gluten free diet – recovery of villous atrophy in three months.

Whipple's disease

1 Infection with *Tropheryma whippelii* (Gram-positive actinomycete)
2 Associated with HLA-B27
3 *Clinical features:*
   (a) diarrhoea

   (b) malabsorption
   (c) arthropathy
   (d) lymphadenopathy
   (e) finger clubbing
4 *Diagnosis* is histological – jejunal biopsy shows macrophages containing PAS-postive granules within the villi
5 *Treatment* – penicillin, erythromycin or cephalosporin (long-term treatment recommended).

Causes of villous atrophy

1 Coeliac disease
2 Dermatitis herpetiformis
3 Whipple's disease
4 Hypogammaglobulinaemia
5 Lymphoma
6 Tropical sprue.

Carcinoid tumours

1 Carcinoid tumours are present in 1% of postmortems
2 Carcinoid syndrome (very rare) – liver metastases lead to systemic release of serotonin
3 Tumours arise from enterochromaffin cells in the lamina propria
4 Appendix is most common site (also bronchial, rectal and ovarian)
5 Clinical features:
   (a) flushing of head and upper thorax
   (b) bronchoconstriction
   (c) diarrhoea
   (d) right valvular stenosis (left if an ASD is present or bronchial carcinoid)
   (e) can lead to pellagra due to tumour uptake of tryptophan
6 *Diagnosis:* 5-hydroxyindoleacetic acid (5-HIAA) detected in the urine
7 *Treatment:*
   (a) surgical resection
   (b) embolisation of hepatic metastases
   (c) phenoxybenzamine for flushing
   (d) octreotide
   (e) nicotinic acid
   (f) cyproheptadine ($5HT_2$ antagonist).

VIPoma

1 90% pancreatic origin
2 50% malignant
3 *Clinical features:*
   (a) secretory diarrhoea (large volume > 3 l/day)
   (b) severe dehydration
   (c) hypotension
   (d) abdominal colic
   (e) flushing
   (f) weight loss
   (g) hypokalaemia and acidosis
4 *Diagnosis:* ↑ VIP, ↑ histidine methionine
5 *Treatment:* resection, octreotide (reduces diarrhoea) and
   chemotherapy.

Protein-losing enteropathy

Excessive loss of protein from the GI tract.

1 Causes:
   (a) giant hypertrophy of gastric rugae – Ménétrier's disease
   (b) regional ileitis
   (c) ulcerative colitis
   (d) tropical sprue
   (e) Whipple's disease
   (f) gastric carcinoma
   (g) intestinal lymphangiectasia
   (h) constrictive pericarditis
   (i) hypogammaglobulinaemia
   (j) erythroderma
   (k) allergic gastroenteropathy
2 *Diagnosis:* rate of loss of protein into the intestine measured with
   radiolabelled (^{51}Cr)-albumin
3 *Treatment:* correct underlying cause.

INFLAMMATORY BOWEL DISEASE (IBD)

Crohn's disease

1 Affects any part of the GI tract, from mouth to anus

2 Commonly terminal ileum, colon, anorectum
3 'Skip lesions' of normal mucosa between affected areas.

Pathology

1 Transmural inflammation
2 Non-caseating granuloma (65%)
3 Fissuring ulcers
4 Lymphoid aggregates
5 Neutrophil infiltrates.

Clinical features

1 Abdominal pain (prominent) and fever
2 Diarrhoea ± blood PR
3 Weight loss
4 Anal/perianal/oral lesions
5 Fistulae
6 Stricturing common, resulting in obstructive symptoms
7 Anaemia (iron, B_{12} or folate deficiency).

Associations

1 Increased incidence in smokers (50–60% are smokers)
2 Erythema nodosum (5–10%)
3 Pyoderma gangrenosum (0.5%)
4 Iritis/uveitis (3–10%)
5 Joint pain/arthritis (6–12%)
6 Cholelithiasis
7 Clubbing
8 Depression.

Diagnosis

1 Barium studies:
    (a) cobblestoning of mucosa
    (b) rose-thorn ulcers
    (c) skip lesions
2 Endoscopy and biopsy
3 Isotope leucocyte scans useful to diagnose active small bowel disease.

Complications

1 Fistulae:
   (a) entero-enteral
   (b) entero-vesical
   (c) entero-vaginal
   (d) perianal
2 Carcinoma – slightly increased incidence of colonic malignancy and small bowel lymphoma
3 B_{12} deficiency (terminal ileal disease)
4 Folate deficiency
5 Osteomalacia
6 Abscess formation
7 Amyloidosis.

Ulcerative colitis

1 Always involves rectum and extends confluently into the colon
2 Terminal ileum may be affected by 'backwash ileitis'
3 Remainder unaffected.

Pathology

1 Mucosa and submucosa only involved
2 Mucosal ulcers
3 Inflammatory cell infiltrate
4 Crypt abscesses
5 Loss of goblet cells.

Clinical features

1 Diarrhoea, often with blood and mucus
2 Urgency and tenesmus
3 Weight loss
4 Fever
5 Abdominal pain less prominent than in Crohn's
6 Iron deficiency anaemia.

Associations

1 ↓ Incidence in smokers (70–80% are non-smokers)

2 ↑ Incidence of primary biliary cirrhosis, chronic active hepatitis and sclerosing cholangitis
3 Other systemic manifestations less common than in Crohn's disease
4 Pancreatitis
5 Hyposplenism
6 pANCA (80%).

Diagnosis

1 Barium studies:
   (a) pseudopolyps
   (b) loss of haustral pattern
   (c) featureless shortened colon
2 Sigmoidoscopy and biopsy may be sufficient.

Complications

1 Toxic megacolon (urgent indication for colectomy)
2 Increased incidence of carcinoma – 20-fold after 20 years of disease
3 Preventative colectomy of value
4 Iron deficiency anaemia
5 Fistulae do not develop.

Treatment of IBD

1 5-ASA compounds (sulfasalazine, mesalazine, balzalazide etc.):
   (a) used to treat acute UC and Crohn's in combination with steroids
   (b) reduce relapse (UC only) by 65%
   (c) topical (enema) or oral
   (d) side-effects of sulfasalazine:
      (i) headaches
      (ii) skin rashes
      (iii) marrow suppression
      (iv) folate deficiency
      (v) haemolysis
      (vi) reversible azoospermia
      (vii) orange urine
2 Steroids:
   (a) topical, oral or parenteral
   (b) treatment of flare-up
   (c) not used long-term as they do not prevent relapses, and

side-effects
3 Azathioprine:
   (a) used as a steroid-sparing agent
   (b) reduces relapses (UC and Crohn's)
4 Nutritional support: an elemental diet is effective in inducing remission
5 Surgery:
   (a) recurrence occurs in 30–60% of patients after surgery in Crohn's disease
   (b) surgery in UC (panproctocolectomy) may be curative
6 Antibiotics: metronidazole effective but side-effects limit long-term use
7 TNF-alpha antagonists (infliximab): used in severe IBD and Crohn's fistulae (see page 67).

Extra-intestinal manifestations of IBD

Related to disease activity

1 Erythema nodosum
2 Pyoderma gangrenosum
3 Arthropathy
4 Conjunctivitis
5 Episcleritis
6 Uveitis
7 Thromboembolic disease
8 Gallstones
9 Amyloidosis
10 Hyposplenism
11 Fatty liver.

Unrelated to disease activity

1 Sacroiliitis
2 Ankylosing spondylitis
3 Primary sclerosing cholangitis.

LARGE BOWEL DISORDERS

Causes of lower GI bleeding

1 Haemorrhoids

2 Anal fissure
3 Diverticulosis
4 Lower GI neoplasia (adenomatous polyps, carcinomas)
5 Inflammatory bowel disease (UC/Crohn's)
6 Infective enterocolitis (*Salmonella, Shigella, E. coli*, amoebiasis)
7 Ischaemic colitis
8 Rectal varices
9 Angiodysplasia
10 Meckel's diverticulum
11 Iatrogenic (endoscopy).

Causes of constipation

1 Inadequate dietary fibre
2 Dehydration
3 Functional constipation (IBS)
4 Pregnancy
5 Immobility
6 Neoplasm
7 Diverticular disease
8 Crohn's disease
9 Hypothyroidism
10 Hypercalcaemia
11 Pelvic mass
12 Spinal cord and sacral nerve disease
13 Pudendal nerve damage
14 Parkinson's disease
15 Hirschsprung's disease
16 Chronic pseudo-obstruction
17 Systemic sclerosis
18 Diabetic neuropathy
19 Drugs:
    (a) opiates
    (b) iron
    (c) anticholinergics
    (d) tricylic antidepressants
    (e) calcium antagonists.

Colorectal cancer

1 Second most common cancer in the UK

2 Adenocarcinoma arising from tubular or villous adenomatous polyps
3 Commonest in rectum (30%) and sigmoid (30%)
4 *Risk factors:*
   (a) male sex
   (b) inflammatory bowel disease (especially UC)
   (c) familial polyposis coli (AD)
   (d) hereditary non-polyposis colon cancer (AD)
   (e) diet low in fibre
   (f) diet high in fat and red meat
   (g) cholecystectomy
   (h) alcohol
   (i) ureterosigmoidostomy
   (j) NSAIDs may be protective
5 *Clinical features:*
   (a) weight loss
   (b) altered bowel habit
   (c) abdominal mass
   (d) right-sided:
       (i) iron deficiency anaemia
       (ii) abdominal pain
   (e) left-sided:
       (i) blood PR
       (ii) altered bowel habit
       (iii) tenesmus
6 *Treatment:*
   (a) surgical resection
   (b) radiotherapy (to debulk tumour before surgery)
   (c) adjuvant chemotherapy postop. for Dukes' B and C (fluorouracil)
   (d) carcinoembryonic antigen (CEA) can be used to monitor for recurrence.

Dukes' staging of colorectal cancer

[See Table 18, overleaf]

Irritable bowel syndrome (IBS)

1 *Diagnosis* by Rome criteria:
   (a) three-month history of abdominal pain relieved by defecation, which is associated with a change in bowel frequency and/or

Table 18

Stage	Extent	Five-year survival
A	Confined to mucosa and submucosa	>80%
B	Extends through muscularis propria	60–70%
C	Regional lymph nodes involved	30–40%
D	Distant spread	0%

      consistency of stool
- (b) together with two or more of:
  - (i) altered bowel frequency
  - (ii) altered bowel consistency
  - (iii) altered ease of defecation
  - (iv) passage of mucus
  - (v) sensation of bloating
2 Pain may be reproduced at sigmoidoscopy by insufflation of air and is eased by passage of this air
3 *Treatment* (but no real evidence that any treatment works):
- (a) dietary modification
- (b) ↑ fibre
- (c) antispasmodics
- (d) anticholinergics
- (e) antidepressants
- (f) prokinetic agents
- (g) psychotherapy.

Causes of intestinal pseudo-obstruction

Primary

Idiopathic.

Secondary

Acute

1 Postoperative
2 Liver failure
3 Acute pancreatitis
4 Acute cholecystitis
5 Intestinal ischaemia

6 Retroperitoneal haematoma
7 Metabolic:
   (a) hypokalaemia
   (b) hyper/hypocalcaemia
   (c) hypomagnesaemia
   (d) hypothyroidism.

Chronic

1 Neurological:
   (a) diabetes mellitus
   (b) Hirschsprung's disease
   (c) Chagas' disease
   (d) Parkinson's disease
2 Myopathy:
   (a) dystrophica myotonica
   (b) polymyositis
3 Muscle infiltration:
   (a) amyloid
   (b) systemic sclerosis
4 Other intestinal disorders:
   (a) jejunal diverticulosis
   (b) coeliac disease
5 Iatrogenic:
   (a) anticholinergics
   (b) antidepressants
   (c) phenothiazines
   (d) opiates
   (e) clonidine.

LIVER DISORDERS

Jaundice

Prehepatic causes

1 Congenital hyperbilirubinaemia:
   (a) Gilbert's syndrome
   (b) Crigler–Najjar syndrome type 1
   (c) Crigler–Najjar syndrome type 2

(d) Rotor syndrome
(e) Dubin–Johnson syndrome
2 Haemolysis (see Haematology).

Hepatic causes

1 Alcohol
2 Hepatitis viruses:
   (a) A–E viruses (see below)
   (b) non A–E viruses
   (c) EBV
   (d) CMV
   (e) HIV
   (f) arboviruses
3 Drugs (see below)
4 Primary biliary cirrhosis
5 Autoimmune (lupoid) hepatitis
6 Primary sclerosing cholangitis
7 Wilson's disease
8 Haemochromatosis
9 Alpha-1-antitrypsin deficiency
10 Hepatocellular carcinoma
11 Liver metastases
12 Budd–Chiari syndrome
13 Cryptogenic
14 Obesity/diabetes (non-alcoholic steatohepatitis)
15 Pregnancy (see below)
16 Right heart failure/constrictive pericarditis
17 SLE
18 Scleroderma
19 Schistosomiasis (*Schistosoma japonicum*)
20 Leptospirosis
21 Toxoplasmosis
22 Amoebiasis
23 Malaria
24 Galactosaemia
25 Cystic fibrosis
26 Glycogen storage diseases.

Posthepatic causes

Benign

1 Gallstones in the bile duct
2 Ascending cholangitis
3 Acute and chronic pancreatitis
4 Post-traumatic stricture
5 Sclerosing cholangitis
6 Biliary atresia
7 Choledochal cyst
8 Retroperitoneal fibrosis
9 Haemobilia
10 Helminthic infections
11 Mirizzi's syndrome.

Malignant

1 Pancreatic carcinoma
2 Cholangiocarcinoma
3 Carcinoma of the gallbladder
4 Carcinoma of the ampulla of Vater
5 Carcinoma of the duodenum
6 Hilar lymphadenopathy.

Congenital hyperbilirubinaemia

[See Table 19, overleaf]

Viral hepatitis

[See Table 20, page 155]

Hepatitis B serology (see also pages 241–242)

HBsAg – present in acute infection. If present for more than six months, signifies chronic hepatitis.
HBeAg – present in acute or chronic infection. Signifies high infectivity (absent in precore mutant).
HBcAg – present in acute or chronic infection. Found only in liver tissue; present for life.
Anti-HBs – signifies immunity after vaccination or acute infection.
Anti-HBe – signifies declining infectivity and resolving infection.

Table 19

Syndrome	Genetics	Defect	Clinical features	Treatment
Gilbert's	AD	Defect in conjugation	Raised unconjugated bilirubin Asymptomatic or jaundice (increases with fasting)	Nil (benign condition)
Crigler–Najjar type 1	AR	Defect in conjugation	Neonatal kernicterus and death	Fatal
Crigler–Najjar type 2	AD	Defect in conjugation	Jaundice as a neonate/child Survive into adulthood	Phenobarbitone reduces jaundice
Dubin–Johnson	AR	Defect in hepatic excretion	Jaundice with RUQ pain and malaise	Nil (benign condition)
Rotor	AD	Defect in uptake and storage of bilirubin	Raised conjugated bilirubin	Nil (benign condition)

Table 20

	Spread	Virus	Clinical features	Treatment	Chronicity	Incubation
A	Faecal–oral	RNA	Anorexia Jaundice Nausea Joint pains Fever	Supportive Benign condition Fulminant hepatitis in 0.2%	No	15–40 days
B	Blood, sexual, vertical	DNA	Asymptomatic jaundice Acute fever Arteritis Glomerulonephritis Arthropathy	Supportive <1% fulminant hepatitis. Chronic HBV may respond to interferon Lamivudine	15–20% (at risk of cirrhosis or HCC)	50–180 days
C	Blood, sexual	RNA	Asymptomatic jaundice Malaise	Fulminant hepatitis rare Chronic HCV may respond to interferon and ribavirin	60–80% (20% risk of cirrhosis and HCC)	40–55 days
D	Blood (dependent on concurrent HBV infection for replication)	Incomplete RNA	Exacerbates HBV infection and increases risk of hepatic failure and cirrhosis	Interferon of limited benefit	Increases incidence of cirrhosis in chronic HBV	
E	Faecal–oral	RNA	Acute self limiting illness In pregnancy mortality (fetal and maternal) of 25 %	Supportive	No	30–50 days

Anti-HBc IgM – signifies recent acute infection. Lasts less than six months.
Anti-HBc IgG – a life-long marker of past acute or chronic infection. Does not signify immunity or previous vaccination.

Primary biliary cirrhosis (PBC)

1 Progressive inflammation and destruction of small bile ducts, leading to cirrhosis
2 Probably autoimmune
3 90% are female
4 *Associations:*
   (a) HLA-DR8
   (b) scleroderma
   (c) CREST syndrome
   (d) Sjögren's syndrome
   (e) seropositve and seronegative arthritis
   (f) thyroiditis
   (g) renal tubular acidosis
   (h) coeliac disease
   (i) pulmonary fibrosis.
5 *Clinical features:*
   (a) asymptomatic
   (b) cholestatic jaundice
   (c) pruritus
   (d) xanthelasma (hypercholesterolaemia)
   (e) skin pigmentation
   (f) clubbing
   (g) hepatosplenomegaly
   (h) portal hypertension
   (i) osteomalacia/osteoporosis
6 *Diagnosis:*
   (a) antimitochondrial antibodies in 95%
   (b) predominantly raised ALP (cholestatic picture)
   (c) raised IgM
   (d) liver biopsy – destruction of interlobular ducts, small duct proliferation, fibrosis and cirrhosis
7 *Treatment:*
   (a) symptomatic therapy
   (b) transplantation

(c) ursodeoxycholic acid may reduce time to transplantation.

Autoimmune (lupoid) hepatitis

1 Female predominance 4 : 1
2 *Associations:* other autoimmune disorders and HLA-DR3 and
   HLA-DR4
3 *Clinical features:*
   (a) can present with an acute hepatitis or with a chronic illness,
        lethargy
   (b) epigastric pain
   (c) arthralgia
   (d) myalgia
   (e) fluctuating jaundice
   (f) cushingoid appearance
4 *Diagnosis:*
   (a) raised IgG
   (b) hepatitic LFTs
   (c) 80% are ANA or SMA positive (type 1)
   (d) 3–4% liver/kidney/microsomal Ab positive (type 2)
   (e) pANCA positive 90%
   (f) liver biopsy is required for diagnosis – interface hepatitis
5 *Treatment:*
   (a) depends on histology
   (b) steroids to induce remission and azathioprine to maintain it.

Primary sclerosing cholangitis (PSC)

1 Obliterative inflammatory fibrosis of the biliary tract
2 Generalised beading of and stenosis of the biliary tract
3 Aetiology unknown
4 *Complications:*
   (a) cirrhosis
   (b) cholangiocarcinoma
5 *Associations:*
   (a) inflammatory bowel disease (mainly UC – 95%)
   (b) HLA-DR2
6 *Diagnosis:*
   (a) ↑ ALP
   (b) bilirubin raised late in disease

(c) ERCP or MRCP for diagnosis
(d) pANCA positive in 80%
(e) smooth muscle antibody (30%)
(f) ANA positive in 30%
7 *Treatment:* symptomatic and liver transplant (second most common reason for transplant in UK).

Hepatocellular carcinoma (HCC)

1 Rare
2 *Predisposing factors:*
   (a) HBV
   (b) HCV
   (c) cirrhosis (any cause)
   (d) aflatoxin (carcinogen from the mould *Aspergillus flavus*)
   (e) long-term OCP use
   (f) thorotrast
3 *Diagnosis:*
   (a) ↑ AFP (80%) > 500 IU/L = high probability
   (b) USS liver
   (c) liver biopsy (can cause seeding of the tumour)
   (d) lipiodol angiogram followed by CT 14 days later can pick up 2–3 mm lesions.

Liver abscess

1 Usually occurs with underlying biliary tract pathology
2 Usually multiple
3 Most frequent organisms are:
   (a) *E. coli*
   (b) *Klebsiella*
   (c) *Proteus*
   (d) *Pseudomonas*
   (e) anaerobes
4 Presents with spiking fevers and RUQ pain
5 *Investigations:*
   (a) ↑ WCC
   (b) ↑ ESR
   (c) abnormal LFTs
   (d) diagnosis on ultrasound or CT

(e) aspiration and culture grows an organism in 90%
6 *Treatment:*
   (a) antibiotics (broad-spectrum and guided by culture results)
   (b) aspiration
   (c) occasionally surgery.

Amoebic liver abscess

1 Caused by *Entamoeba histolytica*
2 Presents with fever and RUQ pain
3 Less than 10% have bloody diarrhoea
4 Usually single
5 More common in the right lobe
6 Diagnosed by USS, CT or serology
7 Aspiration not required (but like 'anchovy paste')
8 Treatment with metronidazole and diloxanide to eradicate luminal organisms.

Hydatid liver cysts

1 Caused by the ingestion of *Echinococcus granulosus* eggs (from dogs and cattle)
2 Eggs hatch in the intestine and migrate to the liver
3 Forms septated calcified cysts (daughter cysts) in the liver
4 Presents with fever, hepatomegaly and eosinophilia
5 Diagnosis with USS, CT and serology
6 Ruptured cysts can cause anaphylactic reactions
7 Treatment with albendazole and surgery.

Causes of Budd–Chiari syndrome

Thrombosis of the hepatic veins.
1 Thrombophilic disorders
2 Tumours:
   (a) HCC
   (b) renal cell
   (c) stomach
   (d) pancreas
   (e) adrenal
3 Drugs:
   (a) OCP

   (b) cytotoxics
4 Infections:
   (a) amoebic abscess
   (b) aspergillosis
   (c) hydatid cysts
   (d) schistosomiasis
   (e) syphilis
5 Trauma
6 Miscellaneous:
   (a) IBD
   (b) nephritic syndrome
   (c) sarcoidosis
   (d) protein-losing enteropathy
   (e) Behçet's disease.

Drugs that cause jaundice

Hepatitis

1 Isoniazid
2 Phenytoin
3 Methyldopa
4 HMG-CoA reductase inhibitors
5 Pyrazinamide
6 Valproate
7 Amiodarone
8 Halothane
9 Methotrexate
10 Diclofenac
11 Busulfan
12 Nitrofurantoin
13 Paracetamol
14 Rifampicin
15 Tamoxifen.

Cholestasis

1 Chlopromazine
2 Carbamazepine
3 Erythromycin
4 Sulphonylureas

5 Oestrogens
6 Anabolic steroids
7 Cimetidine
8 Hydralazine
9 Penicillins
10 Clavulinic acid.

Granulomas

1 Sulphonamides
2 Phenylbutazone
3 Allopurinol.

Malignancy

1 Anabolic steroids
2 OCP.

Fibrosis

1 Methotrexate
2 Vitamin A
3 Retinoids.

Causes of cirrhosis

1 Alcohol
2 Chronic hepatitis B and C virus infection
3 PBC
4 Autoimmune hepatitis
5 PSC
6 Haemochromatosis
7 Wilson's disease
8 Alpha-1-antitrypsin deficiency
9 Intrahepatic biliary obstruction
10 Extrahepatic biliary obstruction
11 Drugs
12 Cardiac failure
13 Budd–Chiari syndrome
14 Obesity/diabetes
15 Sarcoidosis

16 Syphilis
17 Cryptogenic
18 Indian childhood cirrhosis
19 Cystic fibrosis
20 Glycogen storage diseases
21 Galactosaemia
22 Abetalipoproteinaemia
23 Porphyria.

Causes of chronic active hepatitis

1 Hepatitis B
2 Hepatitis C
3 Hepatitis D
4 Autoimmune hepatitis
5 Wilson's disease
6 Haemochromatosis
7 ? Alcohol
8 Drugs (methyldopa, isoniazid, nitrofurantoin).

Causes of hepatic granuloma

1 *Infective:*
  (a) mycobacteria
  (b) brucellosis
  (c) *Yersinia*
  (d) Whipple's disease
  (e) syphilis
  (f) histoplasmosis
  (g) blastomycosis
  (h) *Cryptococcus*
  (i) leishmaniasis
  (j) toxoplasmosis
  (k) schistosomiasis
  (l) EBV
  (m) CMV
  (n) hepatitis A
2 *Metals:*
  (a) beryllium
  (b) copper

3 *Immunological disorders:*
  (a) sarcoidosis
  (b) AIDS
  (c) Crohn's disease
  (d) ulcerative colitis
  (e) PBC
  (f) hypogammaglobulinaemia
  (g) SLE
  (h) polymyalgia rheumatica
  (i) BCG vaccine
4 *Idiopathic:* granulomatous hepatitis
5 *Enzyme defects:* chronic granulomatous disease in children
6 *Neoplasia:*
  (a) lymphoma
  (b) carcinoma.

Clinical signs of chronic liver disease

1 Jaundice
2 Finger clubbing
3 Leuconychia
4 Palmar erythema
5 Spider naevi
6 Bruising
7 Gynaecomastia
8 Testicular atrophy
9 Loss of body hair
10 Ascites
11 Hepatosplenomegaly
12 Encephalopathy
13 Liver flap
14 Caput medusae
15 Peripheral oedema
16 Fetor hepaticus.

Clinical signs of chronic liver disease secondary to alcohol

1 Tremor
2 Parotid enlargement
3 Dupuytren's contracture

4 Pseudo-Cushing's
5 Proximal myopathy
6 Peripheral neuropathy
7 Central neurological signs – Wernicke's encepalopathy/Korsakoff's psychosis
8 Cognitive impairment.

Other effects of alcohol abuse (see also pages 356–357)

Neuromuscular

1 Epilepsy
2 Polyneuropathy
3 Myopathy
4 Withdrawal symptoms.

Cardiovascular

1 Cardiomyopathy (dilated)
2 Beriberi
3 Arrhythmias (AF)
4 Hypertension.

Metabolic

1 Gout
2 Hyperlipidaemia (triglycerides)
3 Hypoglycaemia
4 Obesity.

Respiratory

1 Chest infections
2 TB
3 Aspiration pneumonia.

Haematological

1 Macrocytosis
2 Thrombocytopenia
3 Leucopenia.

Bone

1 Osteoporosis
2 Osteomalacia.

Hepatic encephalopathy

Precipitating factors

1 Infection/spontaneous bacterial peritonitis
2 Oral protein load
3 Upper GI haemorrhage
4 Constipation
5 Diuretic therapy
6 Paracentesis
7 Diarrhoea and vomiting
8 Hypoglycaemia
9 Hypotension
10 Hypoxia
11 Anaemia
12 Sedative/hypnotic drugs
13 Surgery.

Grading

Table 21

Grade	Symptoms and signs
Grade 1	Mild confusion
	Agitation
	Sleep disorder
	Asterixis
Grade 2	Drowsiness
	Lethargy
	Asterixis
	Dysarthria
Grade 3	Somnolent but rousable
	Extensor plantars
	Increased reflexes
Grade 4	Coma

Causes of ascites

1 Venous hypertension:
   (a) cirrhosis
   (b) congestive heart failure
   (c) constrictive pericarditis
   (d) Budd–Chiari syndrome
   (e) portal vein thrombosis
2 Hypoalbuminaemia:
   (a) nephrotic syndrome
   (b) malnutrition
   (c) protein-losing enteropathy
3 Malignant disease:
   (a) secondary carcinomatosis
   (b) lymphoma and leukaemia
   (c) primary mesothelioma
4 Infections:
   (a) tuberculous peritonitis
   (b) fungal (*Candida, Cryptococcus*)
   (c) parasitic (*Strongyloides, Entamoeba*)
5 Miscellaneous:
   (a) chylous
   (b) bile
   (c) pancreatic disease
   (d) urinary
   (e) ovarian disease
   (f) myxoedema
   (g) pseudomyxoma peritonei
   (h) eosinophilic gastroenteritis
   (i) Whipple's disease
   (j) sarcoidosis
   (k) SLE.

Treatments for oesophageal varices

Prophylaxis

Measures to prevent bleeding in patients with known varices:
1 Propranolol
2 Nitrates.

Treatment of bleeding varices

1 Resuscitation
2 Injection, banding and sclerotherapy
3 Octreotide
4 Terlipressin
5 Balloon tamponade (temporary)
6 TIPS
7 Surgical shunt
8 Liver transplant.

Physiological changes in the liver in pregnancy

1 Hepatic blood flow remains constant despite an increase in cardiac output, so proportion of cardiac output is reduced from 35% to 29%, affecting drug metabolism
2 Size of the liver remains constant
3 ALP rises 3–4-fold due to placental production
4 Other biochemistry remains the same.

Liver disease in pregnancy

1 Any liver disease can occur in pregnancy
2 **Hyperemesis gravidarum** – can have abnormal LFTs and jaundice
3 **Intrahepatic cholestasis of pregnancy** – ↑ fetal mortality, 3rd trimester, familial, cholestatic LFTs, resolves with delivery, common, treated with ursodeoxycholic acid.
4 **Acute fatty liver of pregnancy** – 3rd trimester, fulminant hepatitis, immediate delivery required, 20% mortality, rare.
5 **HELLP** – **h**aemolysis, **e**levated **l**iver enzymes and **l**ow **p**latelets, delivery required for treatment
6 **Pre-eclampsia** and **eclampsia** – may lead to fulminant hepatic failure, treatment is delivery.

DISORDERS OF THE PANCREAS

Acute pancreatitis

Causes

1 Gallstones

2 Alcohol
3 Trauma
4 Post-ERCP/surgery
5 Viral (mumps, Coxsackie B, HIV)
6 Hyperlipidaemia
7 Hypercalcaemia
8 Autoimmune (PAN)
9 Hypothermia
10 Scorpion venom
11 Drugs (azathioprine, steroids, furosemide (frusemide), oral contraceptive pill, valproate, didanosine)
12 Idiopathic.

Prognosis

Modified Glasgow prognostic score (validated for gallstones and alcohol) – worse prognosis if >3 of these are present:
1 WCC $> 15 \times 10^9/l$
2 Glucose > 10 mmol/l
3 LDH > 600 U/l
4 AST > 200 U/l
5 Urea > 16 mmol/l
6 Calcium < 2 mmol/l
7 Albumin < 32 g/l
8 $P_a O_2 < 8$ kPa.

Complications

Early

1 ARDS
2 ARF
3 DIC
4 Jaundice
5 Anaemia
6 Hypocalcaemia
7 Hypoalbuminaemia
8 Hyperglycaemia
9 Metabolic acidosis.

Late

1 Abscess
2 Pseudocyst
3 Chronic pancreatitis
4 Diabetes mellitus
5 Pancreatic ascites
6 Splenic vein thrombosis
7 Subcutaneous fat necrosis – Weber–Christian disease.

Causes of raised amylase

1 Acute pancreatitis
2 Pancreatic ascites
3 Pseudocyst
4 Pancreatic fistulae
5 Pancreatic carcinoma
6 ERCP
7 Abdominal perforation
8 Mesenteric infarction
9 Cholecystitis/cholangitis
10 Salpingitis/ectopic pregnancy
11 Acute and chronic hepatocellular disease
12 Ovarian neoplasm
13 Salivary adenitis
14 End-stage renal disease
15 Anorexia
16 Burns
17 Metabolic disturbance.

Chronic pancreatitis

Causes

1 Alcohol
2 Cystic fibrosis
3 Duct strictures
4 Hypercalcaemia
5 Hyperlipidaemia
6 Hereditary

7 Tropical pancreatitis
8 Idiopathic.

Clinical features

1 Chronic severe pain
2 Weight loss
3 Diabetes
4 Malabsorption.

Investigations

1 Calcification on AXR
2 ERCP/MRCP – dilated distorted duct with loss of side-branches
3 CT.

Treatment

1 Pancreatic enzyme supplements
2 Analgesia
3 Stop alcohol
4 Surgery.

MISCELLANEOUS

GI problems in HIV (see also page 6)

Infections

1 Mouth/oesophagus:
   (a) candidiasis
   (b) HSV
   (c) CMV
   (d) oral hairy leukoplakia.
2 Small bowel/colon:
   (a) parasites:
      (i) amoebiasis
      (ii) *Giardia*
      (iii) *Cryptosporidium*

    (iv) *Isospora belli*
    (v) *Microsporum*
    (vi) *Cyclospora cayetanensis*
  (b) viruses:
    (i) CMV
    (ii) HSV
    (iii) adenovirus
  (c) bacteria:
    (i) *Salmonella*
    (ii) *Campylobacter*
    (iii) *Mycobacterium avium intracellulare.*

Neoplasia

1 Kaposi's sarcoma
2 Lymphoma
3 Squamous cell carcinomas.

Causes of calcification on abdominal X-rays

1 Faecoliths
2 Phleboliths
3 Calcified lymph nodes
4 Calcified blood vessels
5 Calculi (renal, gallbladder, prostatic)
6 Calcified pancreas, adrenals, liver, kidney, aorta, psoas muscle or costal cartilage
7 Calcified tumour (dermoid, fibroid, teratoma)
8 Fetus
9 Calcification in the abdominal wall.

Uncommon causes of abdominal pain

1 Gastric dilatation
2 Migraine
3 Epilepsy
4 Lead poisoning
5 Tabes dorsalis
6 Acute intermittent porphyria
7 Addison's disease
8 Haemochromatosis

9 Haemolytic crisis
10 Henoch–Schönlein purpura
11 Hepatoma
12 Hyperparathyroidism
13 Uraemia
14 Intestinal parasites.

Genetics

SINGLE GENE DISORDERS

Autosomal dominant inheritance

1 Achondroplasia
2 Acute intermittent porphyria
3 Adult polycystic kidney disease
4 α_1-Antitrypsin deficiency
5 Ehlers–Danlos syndrome
6 Facio-scapulo-humeral dystrophy
7 Gilbert's syndrome
8 Hereditary spherocytosis
9 Huntington's chorea
10 Hyperlipidaemia type II (familial hypercholesterolaemia)
11 Malignant hyperthermia
12 Marfan's syndrome
13 Myotonia congenita
14 Myotonic dystrophy
15 Neurofibromatosis
16 Noonan's syndrome
17 Osteogenesis imperfecta
18 Polyposis coli
19 Retinoblastoma gene
20 Rotor syndrome
21 Tuberose sclerosis
22 von Willebrand's disease.

Neurofibromatosis

Type 1

1 Over six *café-au-lait* spots

2 Lisch nodules on the iris
3 Peripheral neurofibromas
4 Axillary/inguinal freckling
5 Gene localised to chromosome 17.

Type 2

1 Bilateral acoustic neuromas
2 Other cranial and spinal tumours
3 Lens opacities
4 Peripheral schwannomas
5 Less peripheral neurofibromatosis
6 Fewer than six *café-au-lait* spots
7 Gene localised to chromosome 22.

Autosomal recessive inheritance

1 Albinism (oculocutaneous)
2 Ataxia telangiectasia
3 Congenital adrenal hyperplasia
4 Crigler–Najjar syndrome type I
5 Cystic fibrosis
6 Cystinuria
7 Deafness (some forms)
8 Dubin–Johnson syndrome
9 Familial Mediterranean fever
10 Fanconi's anaemia
11 Friedreich's ataxia
12 Galactosaemia
13 Gaucher's disease
14 Glycogen storage diseases
15 Haemochromatosis
16 Homocystinuria
17 Hurler's syndrome
18 Limb girdle muscular dystrophy
19 Niemann–Pick disease
20 Pendred's syndrome
21 Phenylketonuria
22 Sickle cell disease
23 Tay–Sachs disease

24 Thalassaemias
25 Wilson's disease.

Cystic fibrosis (see also pages 368–369)

1 Gene product is known as the 'cystic fibrosis transmembrane regulator' (CFTR)
2 ΔF508 mutation (a three-base deletion removing a phenylalanine residue from the coding region)
3 *CFTR* gene localised to chromosome 7q.

X-linked inheritance

Recessive

1 Agammaglobulinaemia
2 Becker's muscular dystrophy
3 Chronic granulomatous disease
4 Colour blindness
5 Complete testicular feminisation
6 Duchenne muscular dystrophy
7 Fabry's disease
8 Glucose-6-phosphate dehydrogenase deficiency
9 Haemophilia A (factor VIII)
10 Haemophilia B (factor IX)
11 Hunter's syndrome
12 Hypoxanthine-guanine-phosphoribosyl transferase deficiency
13 Ichthyosis (steroid sulphatase deficiency)
14 Lesch–Nyhan syndrome
15 Nephrogenic diabetes insipidus
16 Ocular albinism
17 Retinitis pigmentosa
18 Wiskott–Aldrich syndrome.

Dominant

Vitamin D-resistant rickets.

Trinucleotide repeat mutations

Repeat units of three nucleotides occur in these single gene defects. The number of repeats varies and may increase in successive generations,

leading to greater severity and earlier onset of disease symptoms ('anticipation'). Examples are:
1 Huntington's disease
2 Spinocerebellar ataxia
3 Spinobulbar muscular atrophy
4 Myotonic dystrophy
5 Friedreich's ataxia
6 Fragile X syndrome.

HISTOCOMPATIBILITY ANTIGENS – THE HLA SYSTEM

1 Situated on the short arm of chromosome 6
2 Class I genes:
    (a) three loci – A, B and C
    (b) class I antigens are expressed on most nucleated cells
    (c) gene products are CD8 receptors
3 Class II genes:
    (a) loci – DP, DQ and DR
    (b) class II antigens are expressed on B lymphocytes, macrophages, activated T lymphocytes
    (c) gene products are CD4 receptors.

HLA disease associations

[See Table 22, opposite]

CHROMOSOMAL ABNORMALITIES

Mechanisms

1 *Translocation:* part of one chromosome is transferred to another non-homologous chromosome (e.g. part of chromosome 21 transferred to chromosome 15, leading to Down's syndrome).
2 *Non-disjunction:* chromosomes fail to separate during meiosis and one zygote has either three homologous chromosomes (e.g. trisomy 21 or Down's syndrome) or only one chromosome (e.g. Turner's syndrome – XO).

Table 22

Disease	Antigen	Relative risk
Idiopathic haemochromatosis	A3	8
Behçet's syndrome	B5	6
Ankylosing spondylitis	B27	87
Reiter's syndrome	B27	37
Subacute thyroiditis	B35	14
Narcolepsy	DR2	50
Goodpasture's syndrome	DR2	16
Multiple sclerosis	DR2	4
Dermatitis herpetiformis	DR3	15
Coeliac disease	DR3	11
Idiopathic membranous nephropathy	DR3	12
Sjögren's syndrome	DR3	10
SLE	DR3	6
Addison's disease	DR3	6
Graves' disease	DR3	4
IDDM	DR3	2
Myasthenia gravis	DR3	2
IDDM	DR4	6
Rheumatoid arthritis	DR4	4
Pernicious anaemia	DR5	5

GENETICS

Klinefelter's syndrome (47,XXY)

1 Affects 1 in 600 males
2 Tall stature
3 Hypogonadism
4 Azoospermia
5 Low IQ
6 Testosterone 50% normal level.

Turner's syndrome (45,XO)

1 Affects 1 in 2500 females
2 Streak ovaries
3 Short stature
4 Hypogonadism
5 Osteoporosis
6 Webbed neck

7 Widely spaced nipples
8 Renal abnormalities (e.g. horseshoe kidney)
9 Coarctation of aorta (10–15%)
10 Normal IQ.

Triple X syndrome (47,XXX)

1 Tall stature
2 Reduced intelligence
3 Mild developmental and behavioural difficulties.

Down's syndrome (trisomy 21)

1 in 700 live births. More common as maternal age increases.

Features

1 Brachycephaly
2 Protruding tongue
3 Single palmar crease
4 Clinodactyly fifth finger
5 Up-slanting palpebral fissures
6 Epicanthic folds prominent
7 Brushfield's spots on the iris
8 Moderate mental retardation.

Associated conditions

There is an increased incidence of:
1 Cardiovascular malformation, e.g. ASD, VSD
2 Haematological abnormalities – ALL, AML
3 GI abnormalities, e.g. Hirschsprung's disease
4 Hypothyroidism
5 Cataracts
6 Early-onset Alzheimer's disease.

Edwards' syndrome (trisomy 18)

1 Characteristic facies
2 Prominent occiput
3 Overlapping fingers

4 Rocker-bottom feet
5 Congenital heart disease
6 Dislocated hips
7 Renal abnormalities
8 Mental retardation.

Patau's syndrome (trisomy 13)

1 Microcephaly
2 Cleft lip and palate
3 Polydactyly
4 CNS abnormalities
5 Congenital heart disease
6 Rectal abnormality
7 Mental retardation.

MITOCHONDRIAL CHROMOSOME DISORDERS

Maternally inherited.
1 Mitochondrial encephalomyopathy, lactic acidosis and stroke-like episodes (MELAS)
2 Myoclonic epilepsy with ragged red fibres (MERRF)
3 Leber's optic atrophy
4 Diseases in which mitochondrial DNA abnormalities have been observed:
  (a) Alzheimer's disease
  (b) diabetes
  (c) Parkinson's disease
  (d) deafness.

Haematology

ANAEMIA

Features

1 Pallor
2 Increased cardiac output, leading to:
    (a) angina
    (b) flow murmurs
    (c) palpitations
    (d) cardiac failure
3 Decreased oxygen-carrying capacity, leading to:
    (a) lethargy
    (b) breathlessness on exertion.

Classification

Anaemia may be classified as:
1 Macrocytic – larger erythrocytes
2 Microcytic – smaller erythrocytes
3 Normocytic – normal-sized erythrocytes.

[See Table 23, overleaf]

Causes of microcytosis

1 Iron deficiency anaemia (IDA) – characteristic pencil cells, ↓ serum iron, ↑ TIBC and ↓ ferritin changes
2 Thalassaemia trait – Mediterranean/Asian origin. Check for Hb A_2 level (raised)
3 Anaemia of chronic disease – underlying disease is normally obvious
4 Sideroblastic anaemia – MCV may be increased, decreased or normal
5 Aluminium toxicity – can occur with haemodialysis.

Table 23

	Microcytic hypochromic	Normocytic normochromic	Macrocytic
Red cell indices	MCV < 80 fl MCH < 27 pg	MCV 80–95 fl MCH > 26 pg	MCV > 95 fl
Causes	Iron deficiency	Many haemolytic anaemias	*Megaloblastic:* Vitamin B_{12} or folate deficiency
	Thalassaemia Anaemia of chronic disease (some cases)	Secondary anaemia Acute blood loss	*Normoblastic:* Alcohol Liver disease Myelodysplasia Aplastic anaemia
	Lead poisoning Sideroblastic anaemia	Mixed deficiencies Bone marrow failure, e.g. post-chemotherapy, infiltration by carcinoma	Myxoedema Reticulocytosis Cytotoxic drugs Pregnancy Myeloma

Causes of iron deficiency

1 Chronic blood loss:
   (a) uterine
   (b) gastrointestinal:
      (i) peptic ulcer
      (ii) hiatus hernia
      (iii) oesophageal varices
      (iv) partial gastrectomy
      (v) carcinoma (stomach, colon, rectum)
      (vi) hookworm infection
      (vii) angiodysplasia
      (viii) colitis
      (ix) piles
      (x) diverticulosis
   (c) uncommon causes of blood loss – haemoglobinuria, haematuria, haemosiderosis, self-inflicted blood loss
2 Increased demands:
   (a) prematurity
   (b) growth
   (c) pregnancy
3 Malabsorption:
   (a) gastrectomy
   (b) coeliac disease
4 Poor diet.

Causes of macrocytosis

With megaloblastic bone marrow

1 Folate deficiency
2 B_{12} deficiency (pernicious anaemia)
3 Drugs, e.g. methotrexate, hydroxyurea, azathioprine.

With normoblastic bone marrow

1 Liver disease
2 Pregnancy
3 Alcohol
4 Myxoedema
5 Reticulocytosis.

With associated haematological diseases

1 Myeloma – raised ESR, leucoerythroblastic blood picture, paraproteins
2 Myelodysplasias – monocytosis, dysplastic morphology, cytopenias
3 Aplastic anaemia – pancytopenia with hypocellular bone marrow
4 Myeloproliferative disorders – polycythaemia rubra vera, essential thrombocythaemia, myelofibrosis, chronic myeloid leukaemia (CML).

Abnormalities of red cell morphology (poikilocytosis)

Table 24

Abnormality	Cause
Tear drops	Myelofibrosis
Helmet cells and fragmented cells	Microangiopathic haemolysis
Pencil cells	IDA (with hypochromic microcytes)
Elliptocytes	Hereditary elliptocytosis
Sickle cells	Sickle cell diseases (with target cells)
Spherocytes	Any cause of haemolysis
	Hereditary spherocytosis
Target cells	Liver disease
	Post-splenectomy
	IDA
	Thalassaemias
Polychromasia	Young red cells (implies high reticulocyte count)

Associations with pernicious anaemia

1 Female sex
2 Blue eyes
3 Fair hair and early greying
4 North Europeans
5 Familial
6 Blood group A
7 Vitiligo
8 Myxoedema
9 Hashimoto's disease
10 Thyrotoxicosis
11 Addison's disease
12 Hypoparathyroidism

13 Hypogammaglobulinaemia
14 Carcinoma of the stomach.

Clinical features of a sickle crisis

1 Bone pain – due to bone marrow infarction
2 Sickle dactylitis – infarction of the small bones of the hands and feet
3 Splenic sequestration crisis – occurs in children, with rapid splenic enlargement leading to severe anaemia
4 Pleuritic pain – caused by localised areas of splenic infarction
5 Thrombotic stroke (rare). Requires urgent exchange transfusion
6 Pulmonary infarction-chest syndrome (serious). Requires exchange transfusion
7 Priapism (painful sustained erection). May require surgical intervention
8 Other areas of sickle infarction may cause:
    (a) retinal detachment or proliferative retinopathy may lead to blindness
    (b) placental infarction
    (c) leg ulcers
    (d) avascular necrosis of the neck of femur
9 Aplastic crisis – usually precipitated by parvovirus B19 infection.

Causes of aplastic anaemia

1 Idiopathic – probably autoimmune in most cases
2 Drugs, including gold, phenylbutazone and chloramphenicol
3 Post-hepatitis – hepatotoxic viruses are often also toxic to bone marrow
4 Chemotherapy and radiotherapy.

Causes of sideroblastic anaemia

1 Congenital – rare, pyridoxine-responsive
2 Acquired:
    (a) primary – one of the myelodysplastic syndromes
    (b) secondary – to alcohol, malignancy, drugs (e.g. antituberculous drugs), connective tissue disorders, heavy metal poisoning (especially lead).

Features of haemolysis

1 Elevated reticulocyte count (> 2%)
2 Jaundice – prehepatic. Unconjugated (water-insoluble) bilirubin levels raised in serum but not in urine. Urinary urobilinogen may be raised
3 Abnormal red cell morphology, particularly spherocytes.

Causes of haemolysis

May be classified as intravascular/extravascular or as genetic/acquired.

Intravascular/extravascular classification

Intravascular

1 Immediate transfusion reaction
2 Paroxysmal cold haemoglobinuria
3 Microangiopathic haemolytic anaemia
4 Glucose-6-phosphate dehydrogenase (G6PD) deficiency
5 Infections (especially malaria)
6 Phosphokinase deficiency
7 Paroxysmal nocturnal haemoglobinuria.

Extravascular

1 Warm autoimmune haemolytic anaemia
2 Cold haemagglutinin disease
3 Haemolytic disease of the newborn
4 Hereditary spherocytosis
5 Haemoglobinopathies.

Genetic/acquired classification

Genetic

1 Membrane defects – hereditary spherocytosis, hereditary elliptocytosis
2 Haemoglobin diorders – sickling disorders, thalassaemia
3 Enzyme defects – G6PD and pyruvate kinase deficiencies.

Acquired

1 Immune:
   (a) iso-immune – haemolytic disease of the newborn, blood

transfusion reaction
(b) autoimmune – warm- or cold-antibody mediated
(c) drug-induced
2 Non-immune:
(a) trauma – cardiac haemolysis, microangiopathic haemolytic anaemia
(b) infection – malaria, septicaemia
(c) hypersplenism
(d) membrane disorders – paroxysmal nocturnal haemoglobinuria
(e) liver disease.

Coombs' (antiglobulin) test

Direct Coombs' test – detects antibody on the patient's red cells
Indirect Coombs' test – detects antibody in the patient's serum.

Direct Coombs' test

In the direct Coombs' test the antibody may be:
1 Opsonising – making the erythrocytes attractive to phagocytes
2 Complement-fixing – causing a local enzymatic lysis in the red cell membrane
3 Agglutinating – clumping may be visible in the test tube.

It is used to detect acquired immune causes of haemolytic anaemia.

Indirect Coombs' test

In the indirect Coombs' test the patient's serum is incubated with test red cells bearing different antigen. This test is used frequently as part of the cross matching process, in which the donor's cells are mixed with the recipient's serum.

Causes of 'warm' autoimmune haemolytic anaemia

1 Idiopathic
2 Secondary, to:
(a) SLE and other autoimmune diseases
(b) chronic lymphocytic leukaemia (CLL)
(c) lymphomas
(d) drugs e.g. methyldopa.

Causes of 'cold' autoimmune haemolytic anaemia

1 Idiopathic
2 Secondary, to:
    (a) infections – *Mycoplasma* pneumonia, infectious mononucleosis
    (b) lymphoma
    (c) paroxysmal cold haemoglobinuria
    (d) syphilis (rarely).

Agents that may cause haemolytic anaemia in G6PD deficiency
(see also page 52)

1 Infections and other acute illnesses (e.g. diabetic ketoacidosis)
2 Drugs:
    (a) antimalarials, e.g. primaquine, chloroquine, pyrimethamine
    (b) sulphonamides and sulphones, e.g. co-trimoxazole, dapsone
    (c) other antibacterial agents, e.g. chloramphenicol, nitrofurans
    (d) analgesics, e.g. aspirin
    (e) anthelmintics, e.g. stibophen, nitrodazole
3 Fava beans (favism) and possibly other vegetables.

Microangiopathic haemolytic anaemia (MAHA)

Clinical features

1 Anaemia
2 Helmet cells
3 Fragmented red cells
4 Polychromasia
5 Reticulocytosis.

Causes

1 Disseminated intravascular coagulation (DIC)
2 Haemolytic uraemic syndrome (HUS)
3 Thrombotic thrombocytopenic purpura (TTP)
4 Malignant hypertension
5 Severe pre-eclampsia.

WHITE CELL DISORDERS

Causes of neutrophilia

Neutrophils $> 7.5 \times 10^9$/litre.
1. Bacterial infections, generalised or localised
2. Metabolic disorders – acidosis, uraemia, poisoning, eclampsia
3. Corticosteroid therapy
4. Inflammation or necrosis – MI, trauma, vasculitis
5. Malignant neoplasms
6. Myeloproliferative disorders.

Causes of lymphocytosis

Lymphocytes $> 3.5 \times 10^9$/litre.
1. Acute viral infections – influenza, glandular fever, acute HIV, mumps
2. Chronic lymphocytic leukaemia
3. Thyrotoxicosis
4. Chronic infections – TB, brucellosis, hepatitis, syphilis
5. Other chronic leukaemias and lymphomas
6. Infancy.

Causes of eosinophilia

Eosinophils $> 0.5 \times 10^9$/litre.
1. Allergy – asthma, hay fever, drugs
2. Parasites – ankylosomiasis, ascariasis, toxocariasis, trichinosis, toxocariasis
3. Skin diseases – eczema, psoriasis, dermatitis herpetiformis
4. Neoplasms, especially Hodgkin's disease
5. Tropical eosinophilia
6. Hypereosinophilic syndrome
7. Eosinophilic leukaemia
8. Miscellaneous causes – sarcoidosis, polyarteritis nodosa, eosinophilic granuloma.

Hypereosinophilic syndrome also known as pulmonary eosinophilia syndrome

Clinical features

1. Weight loss

2 Rashes
3 Fever
4 Peripheral neuropathy
5 oedema
6 Cardiac disturbances.

Pathological features

1 Acute arthritis
2 Pericarditis
3 Cardiac mural thrombosis
4 Chronic endocardial fibrosis
5 Pulmonary abnormalities
6 Splenomegaly.

Causes of monocytosis

Monocytes $> 0.8 \times 10^9$/litre.
1 Recovery phase after chemotherapy or radiotherapy
2 Chronic inflammatory disease, e.g. sarcoidosis, Crohn's disease,
   ulcerative colitis, RA, SLE
3 Infections – TB, leishmaniasis, trypanosomiasis, malaria, brucellosis
4 Hodgkin's disease
5 Myelodysplastic syndromes
6 Acute myelomonocytic leukaemias.

Causes of a leucoerythroblastic blood picture

1 Invasion of marrow space by:
   (a) tumour (metastatic carcinoma)
   (b) myeloma
   (c) lymphoma
   (d) osteopetrosis
   (e) storage disease
2 Severe illness:
   (a) severe haemolysis
   (b) massive trauma
   (c) septicaemia.

Causes of neutropenia

Neutrophils $< 1.5 \times 10^9$/litre.

1 Viral infections
2 Idiosyncratic drug reactions, e.g. to carbimazole (see page 57)
3 Collagen diseases, e.g. SLE, RA
4 Myelodysplasia
5 Marrow infiltration
6 After chemotherapy or radiotherapy
7 Hypersplenism
8 Racial, e.g. Afro-Caribbean and Arab races.

CAUSES OF PANCYTOPENIA

1 Aplastic anaemia, including that due to cytotoxic drug therapy
2 Bone marrow infiltration, e.g. by carcinoma, TB, lymphoma
3 Leukaemia, some myelodysplasias, myeloma
4 Hypersplenism, e.g. Felty's syndrome, Gaucher's disease, portal hypertension
5 Megaloblastic anaemia
6 Myelosclerosis
7 Paroxysmal nocturnal haemoglobinuria (occasionally).

HAEMATOLOGICAL MALIGNANCIES

1 Leukaemias, acute and chronic
2 Lymphomas
3 Myelodysplasias
4 Myeloproliferative disorders.

Acute lymphoblastic leukaemia (ALL)

1 Predominantly affects children
2 Remission may be induced with non-myelosuppressive chemotherapy
3 CNS involvement is common
4 Cure rate over 60% with chemotherapy
5 Further classification is by immunological surface markers
6 *Prognostic indicators:*
   (a) height of presenting WCC (blasts)
   (b) age (under one year or over ten years of age do less well)
   (c) sex (males do less well)

(d) cytogenetics
(e) immunophenotype.

Acute myeloid leukaemia (AML)

1 Predominantly affects adults
2 Marrow hypoplasia required to induce remission
3 CNS involvement unusual
4 Cure rate > 30% with chemotherapy
5 Further classified by morphological appearance
6 *Prognostic indicators:*
   (a) cytogenetics
   (b) age (over 60s do worse)
   (c) response to initial chemotherapy.

The French-American-British (FAB) classification of acute leukaemia

1 A morphological classification
2 Mainly used for AML because in ALL immunophenotype has replaced it
3 It depends on the degree of differentiation of the leukaemic cells and whether a recognised tendency to differentiate along one of the myeloid pathways (e.g. monocytic) is present
4 As with any morphological classification it is rather subjective
5 Classified as M0–M7.

The treatment of AML (M3) requires special attention because the disease and its treatment are characterised by acute fibrinolysis/DIC.

Chronic myeloid leukaemia (CML)

1 A disease of middle age
2 Presents with tiredness, weight loss and sweating
3 Splenomegaly present in 90%
4 Complications associated with marked leucocytosis may be found
5 All patients eventually progress to a 'blast crisis' (after one to ten years)
6 Very high white cell counts (100–500 × 10^9/litre)
7 Platelets are low, normal or high
8 High serum B_{12}
9 Massive neutrophilia with leftward shift

10 Philadelphia chromosome present in most patients
11 Marrow hyperplasia, sometimes with increased reticulin.

The Philadelphia chromosome

The Philadelphia chromosome is a small chromosome 22, resulting from
a reciprocal translocation of genetic material between chromosome 9
and chromosome 22. It is present in:
1 90% of patients with CML
2 5% of children with ALL
3 25% of adult patients with ALL
4 1% of patients with AML.

Chronic lymphocytic leukaemia (CLL)

1 The most indolent of the chronic leukaemias
2 Many cases are discovered as an incidental finding
3 The commonest cause of lymphocytosis in the elderly
4 In 95% of cases the lymhocytes are of B-cell lineage
5 Mature-looking lymphocytes and smear cells are seen on the film
6 Progression through lymphocytosis to lymphadenopathy to
   hepatosplenomegaly and marrow failure occurs, though many
   patients may skip stages.

Non-Hodgkin's lymphomas (NHL)

Low-grade lymphomas

1 Relatively mature cells
2 Without treatment these often take an indolent course
3 Local radiotherapy is often effective
4 Single-agent chemotherapy usually used for diffuse disease.

High-grade lymphomas

1 Cells are immature and disease is progressive without treatment
2 Combination chemotherapy used
3 Six-month courses of treatment are usual
4 No benefit obtained from maintenance therapy.

Lymphoblastic lymphomas

1 Cells are very immature and have a propensity to involve the CNS
2 Treatment as for ALL.

Myeloma

A plasma cell neoplasm which produces diffuse bone marrow infiltration and focal osteolytic deposits.

1 Peak age is 70 years
2 Classification is based on the product of the neoplastic cell:
    (a) IgG (55%)
    (b) IgA (25%)
    (c) light chain disease (20%)
3 *Symptoms* include:
    (a) bone pain (especially back, ribs, long bones, shoulders)
    (b) symptoms of renal failure – due to deposition of light chains
    (c) symptoms of anaemia
    (d) infections
    (e) neuropathy
    (f) symptoms of amyloid deposition
    (g) bleeding
4 *Diagnosis:*
    (a) abundant plasma cells in marrow
    (b) monoclonal band in serum or urine or urinary light chains (Bence Jones protein)
    (c) osteolytic bone lesions
    (d) supported by raised ESR, increased calcium, anaemia, 'pepper pot' skull
1 *Treatment:*
    (a) supportive (treatment of bone pain, transfusion, radiotherapy)
    (b) chemotherapy ± autologous bone marrow transplant
2 *Prognosis:* 50% are alive at two years. Worse if haemoglobin is under 7.5 g/dl and urea is over 10 mmol/l at presentation.

Differentiation of myeloma from benign monoclonal gammopathy of unknown significance (MGUS)

Table 25

Myeloma	MGUS
High levels of paraprotein	Low levels of paraprotein
Paraprotein levels rise over time	Paraproteinaemia remains low over period of observation
Other immunoglobulin levels are depressed	Other immunoglobulin levels are normal
Clinical evidence of myeloma	No clinical evidence of myeloma

Myelodysplasias

These are seen more often now as a result of the ageing population and because FBCs are performed more frequently.

Common features

1 More common in the elderly
2 Cytopenias – reduced haemoglobin is the most common, but there may also be a low WCC and low platelets or a combination
3 Dysplastic changes seen in blood and bone marrow, including hypogranular neutrophils, abnormal neutrophil nucleus lobulation, changes in red cell precursors, and mononuclear megakaryocytes
4 Monocytosis – may be found in all but is most marked in chronic myelomonocytic leukaemia (CMML)
5 Propensity to transform into acute myeloid leukaemia. This can be acute but normally takes years
6 Cytogenetic abnormalities as seen in AML
7 Mainstay of treatment is supportive – antibiotics, transfusion, platelet transfusion.

Classification

Table 26

Myelodysplasia	Special features
Refractory anaemia	Dysplastic morphological feature seen, but difficult to distinguish
Refractory anaemia with excess blasts (RAEB)	As above plus increased number of blast cells in marrow (5–20%)
Refractory anaemia with excess of blasts in transformation (RAEB-t)	As above but 20–30% blasts in marrow
Chronic myelomonocytic leukaemia (CMML)	Monocytosis in marrow and blood
Primary acquired sideroblastic anaemia	Ring sideroblasts in marrow

Complications of bone marrow transplant

Early complications

1 Infections – bacterial, fungal, CMV, HSV

2 Haemorrhage
3 Acute graft-versus-host disease (GVHD)
4 Graft failure
5 Haemorrhagic cystitis
6 Interstitial pneumonitis
7 Veno-occlusive disease.

Late complications

1 Infections – especially varicella zoster
2 Chronic GVHD – hepatitis, malabsorption, scleroderma, serous effusions, arthritis
3 Chronic pulmonary disease
4 Cataracts
5 Infertility
6 Second malignancies.

BLEEDING AND COAGULATION DISORDERS

Vascular disorders

Congenital

1 Hereditary haemorrhagic telangiectasia (Osler–Weber–Rendu syndrome)
2 Connective tissue disorders (Ehlers–Danlos syndrome, Marfan's syndrome, osteogenesis imperfecta, pseudoxanthoma elasticum).

Acquired

Vascular disorders may be secondary to:
1 Severe infections:
   (a) septicaemia
   (b) meningococcal infections
   (c) measles
   (d) typhoid
2 Hypersensitivity vasculitis:
   (a) connective tissue disorders (SLE, RA)
   (b) Henoch–Schönlein purpura
3 Drugs:
   (a) steroids

   (b) sulphonamides
4 Miscellaneous causes:
   (a) senile purpura
   (b) Cushing's disease
   (c) easy bruising syndrome
   (d) amyloidosis
   (e) scurvy
   (f) factitial purpura.

Causes of thrombocytosis

Platelets $> 500 \times 10^9$/litre. It is important (but difficult) to distinguish
between 'essential' causes and 'reactive' (or secondary) causes, unless
there are other markers, either of hyposplenism or of a myeloproliferative
disorder (polycythaemia, splenomegaly, basophilia, increased bone
marrow reticulin, cytogenetic abnormality).
   Secondary causes are therefore often treated in order to aid diagnosis.
They include:
1 Bleeding
2 Infection
3 Infarction
4 Iron deficiency
5 Trauma
6 Thrombosis.

Causes of thrombocytopenia

1 Decreased production – marrow failure (leukaemias and
   myelodysplasias), megaloblastosis
2 Excessive destruction:
   (a) immune thrombocytopenic purpura (ITP)
   (b) viral infections
   (c) drugs
   (d) SLE
   (e) lymphoma
   (f) TTP
   (g) hypersplenism
   (h) HUS
   (i) DIC
3 Platelet aggregation – heparin causes this in 5%.

Coagulation cascades

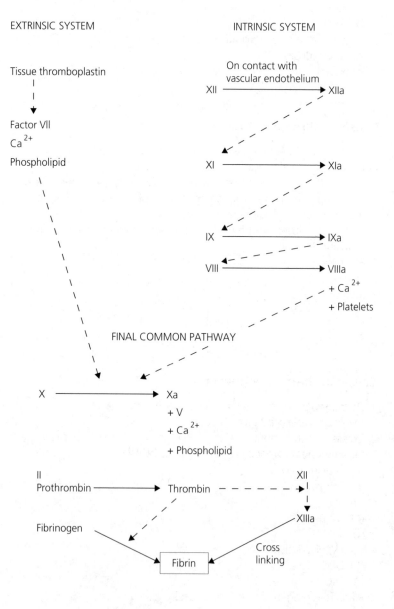

Laboratory coagulation test

1 Prothrombin time (PT) – tests the extrinsic system and the final common pathway
2 Activated partial thromboplastin time (APTT) – a test of the intrinsic and final common pathways
3 Thrombin time (TT) – tests the final part of the common pathway.

Haemophilia A

1 Caused by deficiency of factor VIII
2 X-linked recessive disorder
3 Often presents early in life after trauma/surgery, or with bleeds into joints and muscles
4 Management includes avoiding NSAIDs and intramuscular injections. Minor bleeds – desmopressin, pressure and elevation. Major bleeds (e.g. haemarthrosis) require factor VIII.

Haemophilia B

1 Also known as Christmas disease
2 Caused by factor IX deficiency
3 Behaves clinically like haemophilia A.

von Willebrand's disease

1 Autosomal dominant condition
2 Commonest inherited coagulopathy in the UK
3 The defective gene is on chromosome 12
4 Caused by a quantitive or a qualitative abnormality of vWF (von Willebrand factor) production
5 vWF is made on endothelial cells. It is involved in the adhesion of platelets to damaged subendothelium
6 The disease is usually characterised by mild clinical features, with bruising, superficial purpura, menorrhagia, nose bleeds, and bleeding from cuts and mucous membranes
7 Diagnosis:
   (a) low factor VIII:c
   (b) low vWF: Ag
   (c) prolonged bleeding time
   (d) deficient ristocetin-induced platelet aggregation

8 Treatment is with DDAVP (desmopressin) if mild, and with vWF concentrate.

Disseminated intravascular coagulation (DIC)

1 Caused by release of procoagulant
2 Followed by massive release of coagulation factors and platelets with laying down of fibrin
3 Fibrin is immediately removed as the fibrinolytic system is put into overdrive, worsening the haemmorhagic tendency
4 *Causes:*
   (a) obstetric causes:
      (i) retroplacental haemorrhage
      (ii) retained dead fetus
      (iii) amniotic fluid embolus
      (iv) severe pre-eclampsia
   (b) crush injury
   (c) septicaemia
   (d) haemolytic transfusion reaction
   (e) malignancy
5 *Laboratory results:*
   (a) prolongation of APTT, TT and PT
   (b) increase in fibrin degradation products
   (c) thrombocytopenia
   (d) microangiopathic blood film
6 *Treatment:*
   (a) remove cause
   (b) transfuse with blood, platelets, FFP or cryoprecipitate.

Clinical risk factors for DVT

1 Increasing age
2 Obesity
3 Immobility
4 Varicose veins
5 Previous family history of thrombosis
6 Cancer
7 Major abdominal surgey
8 Trauma to the lower limbs
9 Pregnancy and the puerperium

10 Oestrogen/oral contraceptive pill treatment
11 Increased blood viscosity
12 Nephrotic syndrome
13 Post-MI or stroke
14 Cigarette smoking
15 Diabetic hypermosmolar state
16 Homocystinuria
17 Presence of factor V Leiden mutation
18 Paroxysmal nocturnal haemoglobinuria
19 Protein S, protein C or antithrombin III deficiencies.

Thrombophilia

Indications for investigation

1 Venous thrombosis under the age of 40 years without an obvious
   cause
2 Recurrent venous thrombosis without cause
3 Arterial thrombosis under the age of 30 years without cause
4 Family history
5 Unusual anatomical site.

Causes

Congenital

Deficiencies of :
1 Antithombin III
2 Protein C
3 Protein S
4 Abnormal prothrombin molecule
5 Dysfibrinogenaemia
6 Fibrinolytic defects.

Acquired

1 Polycythaemia and essential thrombocythaemia
2 Lupus anticoagulant/antiphospholipid syndrome.

THE SPLEEN

Causes of splenomegaly

1 Myeloproliferative disorders:
   (a) myelofibrosis
   (b) chronic myeloid leukaemia
   (c) polycythaemia rubra vera
   (d) essential thrombocythaemia
2 Portal hypertension:
   (a) cirrhosis
   (b) congestive cardiac failure
3 Chronic haemolytic anaemias:
   (a) autoimmune haemolytic anaemia
   (b) cold haemagglutinin disease
   (c) hereditary spherocytosis
   (d) haemoglobinopathies
4 Lymphoproliferative disorders:
   (a) most lymphomas
   (b) chronic lymphocytic leukaemia
   (c) hairy cell leukaemia
5 Infections:
   (a) bacterial, e.g. typhoid, *Brucella*, TB
   (b) viral – glandular fever, hepatitis
   (c) protozoal, e.g. malaria, kala-azar
6 Collagen diseases
7 Storage diseases.

Splenectomy

Indications

1 Traumatic rupture – although surgical repair of the capsule is preferable if possible
2 Autoimmune destruction of blood cells – ITP and warm autoimmune haemolytic anaemia after failure of steroids
3 Haematological malignancies – low-grade lymphoproliferative disorders with painful splenomegaly, hypersplenism and limited disease outside the spleen. Also sometimes indicated for myeloproliferative disorders, especially myelofibrosis
4 Congenital haemolytic anaemias – such as hereditary spherocytosis

and hereditary elliptocytosis
5 For staging in Hodgkin's disease and NHL – only done when CT/MRI is unavailable.

Postsplenectomy haematological changes

1 Howell–Jolly bodies – nuclear remnants in red cells, normally removed by the spleen
2 Enhanced neutrophilia in response to infection
3 Target cells, occasionally spherocytes, thrombocytosis
4 Decreased IgM levels.

Causes of hyposplenism

1 Splenectomy
2 Sickle cell disease
3 Coeliac disease
4 Myeloproliferative disorders
5 Congenital asplenism.

Immunology

CELLS OF THE IMMUNE SYSTEM

Polymorphonuclear cells

Neutrophils

1 Multilobed nucleus
2 Half-life of six hours in blood and 1–2 days in the tissues
3 Active in bacterial and fungal infections
4 Stored in bone marrow and released in infections
5 Attracted to infected tissue by:
    (a) cytokines (IL-8, TNF-alpha, GM-CSF),
    (b) bacterial proteins
    (c) leukotrienes (LTB$_4$)
    (d) complement C3b C3a
6 Adhesion molecules (integrins and ICAMs) on endothelium attach to neutrophils and allow them to migrate into the infected tissue
7 Neutrophils pass through endothelium by diapedesis
8 Kill microbes by phagocytosis
9 Oxygen-dependent killing – myeloperoxidase and hydrogen peroxide generate highly reactive oxygen species to kill microbes
10 Oxygen-independent killing involves lysozyme and lactoferrin.

Eosinophils

1 Active against multicellular parasites
2 ↑ in allergic patients
3 Can bind IgE
4 Activated by C3b, C4b, C5a, LTB$_4$, IL-3 and IL-5
5 Migrate like neutrophils
6 Phagocytose Ab–Ag complexes.

Mast cells and basophils

1 Basophils circulate in blood

2 Mast cells are active in the tissues
3 Produce histamine, prostaglandins, leukotrienes and proteases
4 Involved in immune response to parasites
5 Immediate hypersensitivity (type I) caused by interaction with antigen bound to IgE.

Mononuclear phagocyte system

1 Monocytes occur in blood
2 Macrophages active in tissue (Kupffer cells, alveolar macrophages and osteoclasts)
3 Functions:
   (a) cytotoxic (phagocytose opsonised microorganisms – particularly intracellular parasites such as *Mycobacterium tuberculosis*)
   (b) antigen-presenting cells
   (c) produce cytokines:
      (i) IFN-alpha and IFN-beta
      (ii) IL-1
      (iii) IL-6
      (iv) IL-8
      (v) TNF-alpha
   (d) involved in delayed hypersensitivity reactions (Type IV)
   (e) may differentiate to multinucleate giant cells in granuloma.

Lymphocytes

B lymphocytes

1 Mature in bone marrow
2 Form 30% of lymphocytes
3 May differentiate into plasma cells
4 Express MHC class II molecules on surface
5 Express highly specific monoclonal immunoglobulin on surface
6 Mainly activated by IL-4 (IL-2, 5, 6 also involved)
7 Activation requires both antigen and T helper cells
8 When activated there is clonal expansion of the specific B cell, and production of plasma cells and memory cells
9 Plasma cells are non-circulating cells (present in lymphoid organs) that produce specific antibodies
10 Functions:
   (a) antibody production

(b) antigen presentation
(c) production of cytokines to activate T cells.

T lymphocytes

1 Arise from the thymus gland
2 Form 70% of lymphocyte population
3 Important in intracellular infections, tumour surveillance and graft rejection
4 All T cells have CD3 and T cell receptors on their surface
5 Activated T cells also have:
   (a) IL-2 receptors
   (b) transferrin receptors
   (c) MHC class II molecules
6 *T helper cells* (67%):
   (a) have CD4 receptors that interact with MHC class II molecules
   (b) T helper-1 cells:
        (i) involved in cell-mediated immunity
        (ii) activate macrophages
        (iii) activate cytotoxic cells
        (iv) antagonise T_H2 cells
        (v) produce and are activated/influenced by IFN-gamma and IL-2
        (vi) are suppressed by IL-10
        (vii) produce Type IV hypersensitivity
   (c) T helper-2 cells:
        (i) involved in humoral immunity
        (ii) activate and mature B cells
        (iii) antagonise T_H1 cells
        (iv) produce IL-2, IL-4, IL-5, IL-6 and IL-10
        (v) are suppressed by interferons
        (vi) contribute to Type II and III hypersensitivity
7 *T cytotoxic/suppressor cells* (33%):
   (a) have CD8 receptors that interacts with MHC I molecules
   (b) are important in eliminating cells infected with viruses
8 General functions of T cells:
   (a) signalling for B cell expansion and maturation
   (b) recruitment and activation of:
        (i) cells of the monocyte/phagocyte lineage
        (ii) cytotoxic T cells
   (c) secretion of cytokines

(d) regulation of immune reactions.

Natural killer (NK) cells

1 Resemble lymphocytes
2 Kill tumour cells or virally infected cells without prior activation
3 Produce IFN-gamma
4 Activated by IFN-gamma, IL-2, IL-12
5 Cause cell lysis.

Antigen-presenting cells (APCs)

1 Monocytes
2 Macrophages
3 Kupffer cells
4 Dendritic cells
5 Langerhans' cells in skin
6 B lymphocytes.

IMMUNOGLOBULINS

1 Consist of two heavy and two light chains joined by disulphide bonds
2 C region constant
3 V region variable
4 Fab sites bind to antigen
5 Fc site receptor for immune cells.

IgG

1 Monomer
2 Four subclasses – 1 (65%), 2 (20%), 3 (10%), 4 (5%)
3 Most abundant in serum
4 Secondary immune response
5 Can cross the placenta
6 Activates complement via the classical pathway.

IgA

1 Monomer (plasma) or dimer (mucosal surfaces and secretions)
2 Monomer form predominates

3 IgA$_1$ and IgA$_2$
4 Predominantly produced by MALT
5 Activates the alternative pathway
6 A J chain joins the two monomers forming the dimer form
7 Secretory piece facilitates secretion of dimer onto epithelial surfaces.

IgM

1 Pentamer joined by a J chain
2 Primary immune response
3 Very effective agglutinators
4 Opsonises bacteria
5 Includes blood group antibodies.

IgD

1 Monomer
2 Present on B cells
3 Involved in B-cell activation.

IgE

1 Involved in Type I hypersensitivity reactions (anaphylaxis)
2 Present on mast cells and basophils
3 Rises in response to parasitic infections and in atopic patients.

Immunoglobulin levels and age

At birth

IgG: adult levels (active placental transport).
IgA: absent (increased levels suggest acquired *in utero* infection).
IgM: absent (increased levels suggest acquired *in utero* infection).
IgG levels fall at 3–6 months (prone to infection).

Adult levels

IgM: 1 year.
IgG: 5–6 years.
IgA: puberty.

IMMUNOLOGY

COMPLEMENT

1 Postive-feedback enzymic cascade of >40 proteins
2 Complement mainly made in the liver
3 Functions:
   (a) opsonisation and lysis of bacteria
   (b) production of proinflammatory mediators
   (c) solubilisation of antibody–antigen complexes
4 Critical step is activation of C3 to C3b
5 C3 is activated by the classical and alternative pathways
6 *Classical pathway:*
   (a) initiated by Ab–Ag complexes
   (b) components involved: C1q, C1r, C1s, C2, C3, C4
   (c) C4b2a cleaves and activates C3
7 *Alternative pathway:*
   (a) activated by:
      (i) endotoxin
      (ii) bacterial cell walls
      (iii) IgA
   (b) components involved: C3, factor D, factor B and properdin
   (c) C3bBb activates C3
8 *Membrane attack pathway:*
   (a) final common pathway
   (b) generates the more biologically active components such as C5a
     and the membrane attack complex (MAC)
   (c) C5, C6, C7, C8 and C9 involved
9 Important components of the complement pathway:
   (a) C3a:
      (i) mediates inflammation
      (ii) anaphylaxotoxin
   (b) C3b:
      (i) cleaves C5
      (ii) opsonises
      (iii) activates alternative pathway
   (c) C5a:
      (i) mediates inflammation
      (ii) anaphylaxotoxin
      (iii) chemotaxin
   (d) membrane attack complex:

(i) structure that makes holes in cell membranes

(ii) causes lysis of cell membranes and cell death

10 *Regulatory proteins:*

(a) C1 inhibitor: inhibits C1s and C1r irreversibly

(b) C4 binding protein: inhibits cleavage of C3

(c) factor H: inhibits cleavage of C3

(d) decay-accelerating factor (DAF) inhibits cleavage of C3

(e) complement receptor 1: inhibits cleavage of C3.

CYTOKINES

[See Table 27, overleaf]

HYPERSENSITIVITY

Type I – anaphylactic

1 Immediate (< 30 minutes)

2 IgE mediated

3 Specific Ag + IgE + mast cell/basophil = vasoactive mediator release

4 Leads to:

(a) smooth muscle contraction

(b) vasodilatation

(c) increased vascular permeability

(d) attraction of eosinophils

(e) oedema

(f) bronchial constriction

(g) weals

5 Systemic reaction leads to anaphylaxis

6 Local reactions lead to atopy – asthma, hay fever, eczema, allergic rhinitis.

Type II – cytotoxic

1 IgG and IgM antibody mediated

2 Ig + tissue Ag = complement activation, lysis, opsonisation, phagocytosis and inflammation

3 Neutrophils attracted

Table 27

Cytokine	Source	Target cell	Effect
IFN-alpha	Monocytes Macrophages	All	Antiviral ↑MHC expression
IFN-beta	Fibroblasts	All	Antiviral ↑MHC expression
IFN-gamma	T cells NK cells	Macrophages B cells T cells NK cells	Activate Ig class selection Activate and influence T helper type (favours T_H1 cells) Activate
TNF-alpha	Macrophages (main stimulus is bacterial LPS)	Macrophages Neutrophils All cells	Activate ↑cytotoxicity ↑MHC expression Cytotoxic
	T cells	Endothelium T cells	↑adhesion molecule expression Co-signal for activation Cytotoxic
		Other	↑temp via hypothalamus ↑acute phase response via liver
IL-1	Monocytes Macrophages (main stimulus is bacterial LPS)	Endothelium	Pro-coagulant ↑adhesion molecules Co-signal for T-cell activation
		T cells Other	↑acute phase response via IL-6 Induces fever
IL-2	Mainly T_H1 cells	T cells B cells NK cells	Activates cytotoxic T cells (main factor) Growth and differentiation Activate
IL-3	T cells	Immature bone marrow	Promotes growth and differentiation
IL-4	T_H2 cells	T cells	Activate T_H2 cells Inhibits T_H1 cells
		B cells Macrophages	Activator and growth factor Inhibit

Cytokine	Secreted by	Target	Function
IL-5	T$_H$2 cells	Eosinophils	Growth and differentiation Promotes killing of helminthic infections
IL-6	T$_H$2 cells (stimulated by IL-1)	B cells B cells Liver	Growth and differentiation and enhances Ig production Growth factor Acute phase reactant
IL-7	Marrow stromal cells	B cells	Growth and differentiation
IL-8	Monocytes Macrophages T cells Endothelium	Neutrophils	Activation
IL-10	T$_H$2	T cells	Immunosuppressant Inhibits cytokine release and proliferation of T cells
IL-12	T cells B cells NK cells	B cells NK cells T$_H$1 cells	Promotes differentiation Most potent stimulator, enhancing IFN-gamma release by NK cells and cytotoxic activity Activates T$_H$1 cells
TGF-beta	Monocytes CD4 T cells Monocytes Macrophages	CD4 T cells Cytotoxic T cells	Inhibits proliferation Inhibits maturation
G-CSF	CD4 cells T cells Endothelium Monocytes Macrophages	Granulocytes	Promotes growth and differentiation
GM-CSF	CD4 cells T cells Endothelium Monocytes Macrophages	Granulocytes Monocytes	Promotes growth and differentiation

4 Examples:
   (a) transfusion reactions
   (b) haemolytic disease of the newborn
   (c) idiopathic thrombocytopenia
   (d) haemolytic anaemia
   (e) pernicious anaemia
   (f) pemphigus
   (g) myasthenia gravis
   (h) Goodpasture's syndrome
   (i) rheumatic fever
   (j) drug-induced nephritis
   (k) hyperacute allograft rejection.

Type III – immune complex

1 Circulating antibody that reacts with free antigen, forming immune complexes
2 Ig–Ag deposits lead to complement, mast-cell and neutrophil activation
3 Leads to:
   (a) vasculitis (complexes deposited in vessels)
   (b) nephritis (complexes deposited in kidneys)
   (c) extrinsic allergic alveolitis (complexes deposited in lungs)
4 Examples:
   (a) arthrus reaction
   (b) serum sickness
   (c) SLE
   (d) rheumatoid arthritis
   (e) glomerulonephritis
   (f) vasculitis
   (g) subacute bacterial endocarditis
   (h) extrinsic allergic alveolitis
   (i) HSP.

Type IV – delayed hypersensitivity

1 Involves cell-mediated cytotoxicity (CD4 T cells), mediator release and macrophage activation
2 Reaction after > 12 hours
3 Leads to:

(a) erythema
(b) granuloma formation
4 Examples:
(a) TB
(b) Mantoux test
(c) graft rejection
(d) graft-versus-host disease
(e) contact dermatitis.

Type V

1 Antibody reacts with a surface receptor to switch on a cell
2 Graves' disease due to thyroid-stimulating antibodies.

IMMUNODEFICIENCY

Primary B-cell and antibody deficiencies

X-linked infantile (Bruton's) agammaglobulinaemia

1 X-linked
2 Expressed at 5–6 months when maternal derived IgG falls
3 Absent B cells
4 Pre-B cells present in bone marrow but they cannot mature into plasma cells
5 Gene defect on X chromosome leading to absent Bruton's tyrosine kinase
6 Severe depression or absence of all immunoglobulins
7 Lymph nodes small and tonsils absent
8 Recurrent pyogenic bacterial infections (particularly encapsulated organisms)
9 Malabsorption syndrome due to *Giardia lamblia* infection
10 Many live 20–30 years
11 Often die of bronchiectasis
12 Treatment with intravenous gammaglobulin and prophylactic antibiotics.

Selective IgA deficiency

1 Recurrent sinus and respiratory infections

2 Chronic diarrhoeal diseases
3 Increased incidence of coeliac disease
4 Associated with HLA-B8, HLA-DR3 and autoimmune disease (see below)
5 IgA antibodies in 30–40% – may lead to anaphylaxis during blood transfusion
6 20% have IgG subclass (2 and 4) deficiencies – more severe respiratory infections
7 Some patients develop increased IgM (hyper-IgM syndrome)
8 Symptomatic treatment
9 Gammaglobulin only used if there is an associated IgG subclass deficiency.

T-cell disorders

Congenital thymic aplasia (DiGeorge's syndrome)

1 Thymus and parathyroids fail to develop (third and fourth pharyngeal pouches)
2 Defect on chromosome **22**
3 *Clinical features* (**catch 22**):
    (a) **C**ongenital heart disease
    (b) **A**bnormalities of facial and ear structures
    (c) **T**hymic aplasia
    (d) **C**left palate
    (e) **H**ypoparathyroidism/hypocalcaemia/hypothyroidism
    (f) ↓ cell-mediated immunity, leading to:
        (i) chronic rhinitis
        (ii) recurrent pneumonia
        (iii) candidiasis
        (iv) diarrhoea
4 *Treatment:*
    (a) symptomatic (calcium etc.)
    (b) surgery
    (c) thymic transplantation.

Combined B cell and T cell disorders

Severe combined immunodeficiency disease

1 X-linked or AR

2 Failure of stem cells to differentiate into T and B cells
3 Some are caused by lack of adenosine deaminase (AR)
4 Infants have very few lymphocytes in blood or lymphoid tissue
5 Susceptible to all microbial infections, notably rotavirus, CMV, *Candida*, *Pneumocystis carinii*
6 Symptoms occur in early infancy and are fatal in the first year of life if untreated
7 Bone marrow transplant is the treatment of choice.

Common variable immunodeficiency

1 AD/AR
2 Onset 15–35 years
3 Combined B/T-cell defects
4 Impaired cell-mediated immunity
5 ↓ Immunoglobulins (< 3 g/l)
6 May follow EBV infection
7 Associated with IgA deficiency
8 Treatment with intravenous gammaglobulin and prophylactic antibiotics
9 *Clinical features:*
   (a) recurrent pyogenic bacterial infections
   (b) autoimmune diseases common (especially PA)
   (c) increased incidence of *Giardia lamblia* and malabsorption
   (d) lactose intolerance
   (e) anaemia
   (f) splenomegaly
   (g) thrombocytopenia
   (h) lymphoid malignancies
   (i) arthritis
   (j) leucopenia.

Ataxia telangiectasia syndrome

1 AR
2 Failure of DNA repair
3 Deficiencies of T cells, IgA, IgG_2 and IgG_4
4 *Clinical features:*
   (a) cerebellar ataxia (presents at 18 months)
   (b) recurrent sinus/pulmonary infections

(c) oculocutaneous telangiectasia (age six years)
(d) ↑ malignancy
(e) endocrine abnormalities:
  (i) glucose intolerance
  (ii) hypogonadism
  (iii) abnormal liver enzymes
  (iv) ↑ AFP and CEA
5 *Treatment:*
  (a) antibiotics and sunscreens
  (b) immunoglobulins reduce infective episodes.

Wiskott–Aldrich syndrome

1 X-linked recessive
2 Defect in WASP (Wiskott–Aldrich specific protein) gene – impaired intracellular signalling in T cells and failure of T cells to help B cells
3 Normal circulating lymphocyte numbers
4 IgG Normal
5 IgA ↑
6 IgE ↑
7 IgM ↓
8 *Clinical features:*
  (a) thrombocytopenia (severe)
  (b) multiple infections
  (c) eczema
  (d) lymphoid malignancies
  (e) bleeding episodes
  (f) autoimmune disease
9 Treated with bone marrow transplant.

Primary phagocytic disorders

Chronic granulomatous disease

1 AR or X-linked
2 Neutrophils lack the NADPH oxidase necessary to produce highly reactive oxygen species to kill microorganisms
3 Normal numbers of neutrophils
4 Diagnosed by inability of phagocytes to reduce nitroblue tetrazolium dye
5 Leads to granuloma formation

6 *Clinical features:*
   (a) pneumonia
   (b) lymphadenitis
   (c) abscesses (skin, liver, other viscera)
7 Interferon-gamma reduces infection rate.

Leucocyte adhesion deficiency

1 Defect in CD18
2 Leucocytes unable to adhere to vascular endothelium expressing ICAM-1, so cannot migrate
3 Cannot form pus efficiently
4 Present with severe bacterial infections
5 Can be treated with bone marrow transplant.

Chediak–Higashi disease

1 Defects in microtubules lead to inability of lysosomes to release their granules
2 Partial albinism and recurrent pyogenic infections
3 Poor prognosis – most die in childhood
4 Treatment with antibiotics.

Job's syndrome

1 Neutrophils do not respond to chemotactic stimuli
2 Recurrent cold staphylococcal abscesses (boils)
3 Chronic eczema
4 Otitis media
5 ↑ IgE.

Complement deficiency

Primary complement deficiencies

[See Table 28, overleaf]

Hereditary angio-oedema

1 AD
2 85% due to deficiency of C1 esterase
3 15% due to defective C1 esterase

Table 28

Deficiency	Disorder
C1qrs, C2, C4	Immune complex disease
C1 esterase inhibitor	Hereditary angio-oedema
C3, factor H, factor I	Recurrent pyogenic infections
C5–8, properdin, factor D	Recurrent Neisseria infections
C9	Asymptomatic
CD59, DAF, proteins	Paroxysmal nocturnal haemoglobinuria

4 *Clinical features:*
  (a) recurrent oedema:
      (i) subcutaneous (non-itchy, no erythema) – 91%
      (ii) laryngeal (stridor) – 48%
      (iii) intestinal (abdominal pain or obstruction)
  (b) onset in 1–2 hours
  (c) resolves in 24–48 hours
  (d) first attacks usually in childhood
  (e) precipitating factors:
      (i) intercurrent infection
      (ii) stress
      (iii) trauma
      (iv) menstruation
      (v) autoimmune disease
      (vi) ACE inhibitor
      (vii) OCP
5 *Diagnosis:*
  (a) decreased C2 and C4 during an attack
  (b) C3 normal
  (c) decreased C1 esterase
6 *Treatment:*
  (a) intravenous C1 esterase inhibitor/FFP
  (b) prophylaxis with danazol or tranexamic acid.

Paroxysmal nocturnal haemoglobinuria

1 Absence of inhibitors of complement activation (DAF/CD59)
2 Cells susceptible to complement-induced lysis
3 Acquired clonal disorder

4 Leads to intravascular haemolysis
5 Predisposes to venous thromboembolism and infection
6 Can evolve into aplastic anaemia or acute leukaemia
7 *Clinical features:*
   (a) haemoglobinuria
   (b) jaundice
   (c) anaemia
   (d) abdominal pain
8 Diagnosis by Ham's test
9 Treatment supportive with anticoagulation and antibiotics
10 Severe cases may need bone marrow transplant.

Secondary complement deficiencies

Occur in:
1 Post-streptococcal nephritis
2 SLE
3 Chronic membranoproliferative GN
4 Serum sickness
5 Bacterial septicaemia with capsular microorganisms
6 Malaria
7 Liver disease.

Acquired immunodeficiency

Immunoglobulin deficiency

May be due to:
1 Drugs:
   (a) gold
   (b) phenytoin
   (c) penicillamine
   (d) idiosyncratic reactions
2 Haematological malignancy: CLL
3 Protein loss:
   (a) nephrotic syndrome
   (b) protein-losing enteropathy.

Cell-mediated dysfunction

May be caused by:

1 Drugs:
  (a) ciclosporin
  (b) cyclophosphamide
  (c) steroids
2 Haematological malignancy: lymphoma
3 AIDS.

MAJOR HISTOCOMPATIBILITY COMPLEX (MHC)

1 Genes expressed on short arm of chromosome 6
2 Codes for human leucocyte antigens (HLA)
3 HLA are molecules involved in antigen recognition by T lymphocytes
4 T lymphocytes will only recognise antigen that is presented by an HLA molecule
5 *Class I:*
  (a) A, B, C
  (b) present on almost all cells
  (c) signals that carrier cell is 'infected' and suitable for destruction
  (d) only interacts with CD8 cytotoxic T cells
6 *Class II:*
  (a) DP, DQ, DR
  (b) present on B cells, macrophages, dendritic cells and activated T cells
  (c) interacts with CD4 T helper cells to protect against cytotoxic T cells
7 *Class III:* codes for complement C4 and factor B.

TRANSPLANTATION

Types of transplant

1 *Autograft* – transplant within one individual
2 *Syngraft* – transplant between genetically identical individuals
3 *Allograft* – transplant between non-identical individuals
4 *Xenograft* – transplant between species.

Rejection
Table 29

Type	Time	Pathophysiology
Hyperacute	Minutes	Due to preformed antibodies, i.e. ABO mismatch or antibodies to HLA class I molecules from previous transfusion or transplant
Acute	< 10 days	Mediated by CD8 cytotoxic T cells
Chronic	Years	Unclear. Could be due to immune complex deposition and complement activation

Graft-versus-host disease

1 Immunocompetent T cells from the graft recognise alloantigens from the recipient and cause an immune response
2 Relatively common after bone marrow transplant
3 *Clinical features:*
   (a) dermatitis (mild to severe necrolytic)
   (b) diarrhoea (mild to severe)
   (c) cholestatic liver disease
   (d) destruction of red blood cells
   (e) can be fatal
4 Chances reduced by close HLA matching and selective destruction in the T lymphocytes using monoclonal antibodies
5 Treatment with cyclosporin, methyl prednisolone and antithymocyte globulin.

VACCINES

Live attenuated vaccines

1 Measles
2 Mumps
3 Rubella
4 Polio (Sabin)
5 Varicella zoster
6 BCG (TB)
7 Yellow fever.

Inactivated (killed) vaccines

1 Polio (Salk)
2 Influenza
3 Rabies
4 Cholera
5 Typhoid
6 Pertussis
7 Hepatitis A
8 Japanese encephalitis.

Subunit vaccines

1 Hepatitis B
2 Influenza
3 *Streptococcus pneumoniae*
4 *Neisseria meningitidis* types A and C
5 *Haemophilus influenzae* type b.

Preformed antibody vaccines

1 Tetanus
2 Hepatitis B
3 Botulism
4 Rabies
5 Varicella
6 Diphtheria.

Current immunisation guidelines (September 2001)

[See Table 30, opposite]

High-risk groups

1 Hepatitis A
2 Hepatitis B
3 Influenza
4 Pneumococcal
5 Rabies.

Table 30

Age	Vaccines
Two, three and four months	Triple vaccine (diphtheria, tetanus, pertussis) Hib (*Haemophilus influenzae* b) Meningococcal C Polio (BCG in high-risk children)
Twelve to fifteen months	MMR
Four to five years	Polio booster Diphtheria and tetanus booster MMR booster
Ten to fourteen years	BCG
Fifteen to eighteen years	Diphtheria and tetanus booster Polio booster
Adulthood	Rubella in women seronegative for rubella Tetanus ten-yearly

Vaccines for travellers to high-risk areas

1 Yellow fever
2 Typhoid
3 Cholera
4 Hepatitis A
5 Japanese encephalitis.

MISCELLANEOUS

Indications for intravenous immunoglobulin

1 Primary immunodeficiency:
   (a) X-linked hypogammaglobulinaemia
   (b) common variable immunodeficiency
2 Secondary immunodeficiency:
   (a) CLL
   (b) bone marrow transplantation
   (c) paediatric AIDS
   (d) myeloma

3 Inflammatory conditions:
  (a) Kawasaki's disease
  (b) ITP
  (c) Guillain–Barré syndrome.

The acute phase response

1 Normocytic anaemia
2 ↑ Immunoglobulins
3 CRP
4 Serum amyloid P component (AP)
5 Mannose-binding protein
6 Ferritin
7 ↑ Fibrinogen leads to ↑ ESR
8 ALP
9 ↓ Albumin
10 ↑ Platelets
11 ↑ Complement
12 ↑ Caeruloplasmin
13 ↑ Alpha-1 antitrypsin
14 ↑ Angiotensin
15 ↑ Haptoglobin
16 ↑ Fibronectin.

C-reactive protein (CRP)

1 Useful in monitoring inflammation
2 Acute phase reactant
3 Rises within hours
4 Falls in 2–3 days
5 Marked elevation in:
  (a) bacterial infection
  (b) abscess
  (c) Crohn's disease
  (d) connective tissue diseases (except SLE)
  (e) neoplasia
  (f) trauma
  (g) necrosis
6 Normal or slight elevation in:
  (a) viral infection

(b) steroids/oestrogens
(c) ulcerative colitis
(d) SLE.

Autoantibodies in autoimmune disease

Table 31

Disease	Antigen
Hashimoto's thyroiditis	Thyroglobulin
	Thyroid peroxidase
Graves' disease	TSH receptor
Pernicious anaemia	Intrinsic factor
	Parietal cell
Addison's disease	Adrenal cortex cells (17/21 hydroxylase)
Insulin-dependent diabetes mellitus	Cytoplasm of islet cells
	Insulin
	Glutamic acid decarboxylase (GAD) – also in stiff-man syndrome
Myasthenia gravis	Acetylcholine receptor
Lambert–Eaton syndrome	Calcium channels on nerve endings
Gullain–Barré syndrome	Peripheral nerve myelin components
Paraneoplastic polyneuropathies	CNS proteins – Hu, Yo, Ri
Goodpasture's syndrome	Glomerular and lung basement membrane
Pemphigoid	Skin basement membrane
Pemphigus	Desmosomes between prickle cells in epidermis
Autoimmune haemolytic anaemia	Erythrocytes
Idiopathic thrombocytopenia	Platelets
Primary biliary cirrhosis	Mitochondria
Chronic active hepatitis	ANA
	Smooth muscle
	Liver/kidney/ microsomal
Some male infertility	Spermatozoa

Autoantibodies in rheumatological disorders – see Rheumatology.

Autoimmune polyglandular syndromes

Type 1

1 Mucocutaneous candidiasis

2 Adrenal failure
3 Hypoparathyroidism
4 Gonadal failure
5 Alopecia
6 Malabsorption
7 Autoimmune hepatitis.

Type 2

1 Adrenal failure
2 Thyroid disease
3 Type 1 diabetes
4 Gonadal failure
5 Vitiligo
6 Coeliac disease
7 Myasthenia gravis.

Eicosanoids

Prostaglandins

1 Produced by cyclooxygenase from arachidonic acid
2 PGI_2:
   (a) prostacyclin
   (b) produced in vascular endothelium
   (c) causes vasodilatation
   (d) inhibits platelet aggregation
3 PGD_2:
   (a) mainly produced in mast cells
   (b) produces vasodilatation and oedema
4 PGE_2:
   (a) causes vasodilatation and oedema
   (b) ↑ pain
   (c) ↑ fever
5 $PGF_{2\alpha}$: causes vasodilatation and oedema
6 Thromboxane A_2:
   (a) produced in platelets
   (b) causes platelet aggregation
   (c) vasoconstrictor.

Leukotrienes

1 Produced by lipoxygenase from arachidonic acid in neutrophils
2 LTB_4:
   (a) potent chemotactic factor
   (b) aggregates neutrophils
3 LTC_4, D_4, E_4:
   (a) vasoconstrict
   (b) cause bronchospasm
   (c) increase vascular permeability.

Infectious Diseases

MODES OF TRANSMISSION OF INFECTIOUS DISEASES

1 Airborne (measles, diphtheria, tonsillitis, whooping cough, tuberculosis)
2 Intestinal (enterovirus infection, viral hepatitis, poliomyelitis, salmonellosis, Q fever)
3 Direct contact (impetigo, scabies)
4 Venereal (gonorrhoea, syphilis)
5 Insect or animal bites (malaria, leishmaniasis, trypanosomiasis, rabies)
6 Parenteral (HIV, hepatitis B, hepatitis C)
7 Congenital.

FACTORS AFFECTING VULNERABILITY TO INFECTIOUS DISEASE

1 Immunological:
   (a) genetic deficiency (immunoglobulin/complement/T-cell deficiencies)
   (b) prior immunity (natural or vaccine-related)
   (c) acquired deficiency (HIV, malignant disease, transplant patients)
   (d) miscellaneous (diabetes, pregnancy, splenectomy)
2 Psychological status
3 Nutritional status
4 The presence of foreign bodies
5 Behavioural factors (smoking, alcoholism)
6 Previous antibiotics (e.g. MRSA, *Clostridium difficile*).

231

NOTIFIABLE DISEASES (UK)

Acute encephalitis
Acute poliomyelitis
Anthrax
Cholera
Dysentery (amoebic or bacillary)
Ebola
Food poisoning
Diphtheria
Leprosy
Leptospirosis
Malaria
Measles
Meningitis
Meningococcal septicaemia
Mumps

Ophthalmia neonatorum
Paratyphoid fever
Plague
Rabies
Relapsing fever
Scarlet fever
Smallpox
Tetanus
Tuberculosis
Typhoid fever
Viral haemorrhagic fever
Viral hepatitis
Whooping cough
Yellow fever.

VACCINATION

Contraindications to vaccination

1 Untreated malignant disease
2 Patients receiving immunosuppressive treatment
3 Pregnancy
4 Within three weeks of being given another live vaccine
5 Coincidental severe febrile illness
6 Rubella not to be given in pregnancy. Pregnancy should be avoided for up to one month after vaccination.

Types of vaccine

1 Inactivated/killed (predominantly bacterial)
   (a) toxoids (diphtheria, tetanus)
   (b) killed cell (pertussis, typhoid)
   (c) capsular polysaccharide (*Haemophilus influenzae* b, meningococcus, pneumococcus)
2 Attenuated/live (predominantly viral)
   (a) attenuated (measles, mumps, rubella, yellow fever, polio)
   (b) subunit (hepatitis B)

(c) inactivated (rabies, Japanese encephalitis, influenza, hepatitis A)

3 Attenuated bacterial vaccines (BCG, oral typhoid vaccine).

British vaccination schedule
Table 32

Age	Vaccines
Two, three and four months	Triple vaccine (diphtheria, tetanus, pertussis)
	Hib (*Haemophilus influenzae* b)
	Meningococcal C
	Polio
	(BCG in high-risk children)
Twelve to fifteen months	MMR
Four to five years	Polio booster
	Diphtheria and tetanus booster
	MMR booster
Ten to fourteen years	BCG
Fifteen to eighteen years	Diphtheria and tetanus booster
	Polio booster
Adulthood	Rubella in women seronegative for rubella
	Tetanus ten-yearly

ANTIMICROBIAL DRUGS

Choice of antibiotic

1 Blind therapy:
   (a) based on clinical diagnosis
   (b) based on geographical location
   (c) if awaiting microbiological sensitivities
2 Spectrum of activity: should be as narrow as possible, although blind prescribing leads to greater use of broad-spectrum antibiotics
3 Bactericidal *versus* bacteristatic?: no firm evidence, but bactericidal drugs should be used in bacterial endocarditis
4 Patient factors:
   (a) site of infection (brain, eye and loculated abscesses are inaccessible)
   (b) renal/hepatic impairment.

Types of antibiotics

1 Inhibitors of cell wall synthesis:

   (a) β-lactams:
      (i) penicillins (benzyl penicillin, ampicillin, piperacillin)
      (ii) cephalosporins (cefalexin, cefotaxime)
      (iii) monobactams (aztreonam)
      (iv) carbapenems (imepenem)
   (b) glycopeptides (vancomycin, teicoplanin)
2 Inhibitors of protein synthesis:
   (a) macrolides (erythromycin, azithromycin, clarithromycin)
   (b) aminoglycosides (gentamicin, tobramycin, amikacin)
   (c) tetracycyline
   (d) chloramphenicol
   (e) clindamycin
   (f) fusidic acid
3 Inhibitors of DNA replication:
   (a) quinolones
   (b) metronidazole
4 Inhibitors of folate synthesis (e.g. co-trimoxazole).

Bactericidal antibiotics

1 Penicillins
2 Cephalosporins
3 Aminoglycosides.

Antituberculous drugs

1 Rifampicin – inhibits DNA-dependent RNA polymerase
2 Isoniazid – inhibits cell wall synthesis
3 Pyrazinamide – poorly understood, probably works inside phagosomes
4 Ethambutol – inhibits bacterial RNA synthesis
5 Streptomycin – inhibits bacterial protein synthesis.

Antiviral drugs (non-HIV)

1 Aciclovir – active against herpes simplex virus and varicella zoster virus
2 Ganciclovir – as above but also against cytomegalovirus (CMV)
3 Ribavirin – used in aerosol against respiratory syncytial virus (RSV); also for hepatitis C with interferon; Lassa fever (has to be early).

Anthelmintic drugs

1 Benzimidazoles (albendazole, tiabendazole, mebendazole), used for:
   (a) *Trichuris*
   (b) hookworms
   (c) *Enterobius*
   (d) *Ascaris*
   (e) *Taenia*
   (f) *Echinococcus*
2 Piperazines, used for:
   (a) *Ascaris*
   (b) *Enterobius*
3 Diethylcarbamazine (DEC), for: microfilarial disease (*Onchocerca volvulus, Wuchereria bancrofti, Brugia malayi*)
4 Praziquantel, for:
   (a) *Schistosoma*
   (b) *Taenia.*

CAUSES OF PYREXIA OF UNKNOWN ORIGIN (PUO)

1 Infection (35%):
   (a) TB
   (b) hidden abscesses
   (c) subacute bacterial endocarditis
   (d) infectious mononucleosis
   (e) CMV infection
   (f) brucellosis
   (g) chronic prostatitis
2 Neoplasia (25%):
   (a) Hodgkin's disease and other lymphomas
   (b) leukaemias
   (c) solid tumours (renal, pancreatic, hepatocellular)
   (d) metastatic carcinoma
3 Connective tissue disease (20%):
   (a) rheumatoid
   (b) SLE
   (c) PAN
4 Miscellaneous causes (15%):
   (a) sarcoid
   (b) multiple pulmonary emboli

(c) Crohn's disease
(d) familial Mediterranean fever
(e) drugs
5 Undiagnosed (5–10%).

MEDICALLY IMPORTANT GRAM-POSITIVE BACTERIA

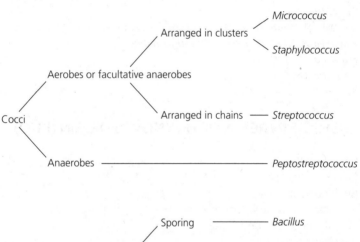

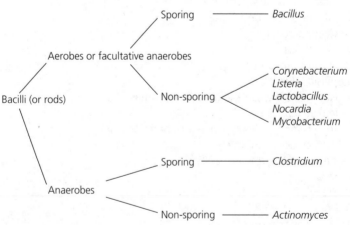

MEDICALLY IMPORTANT GRAM-NEGATIVE BACTERIA

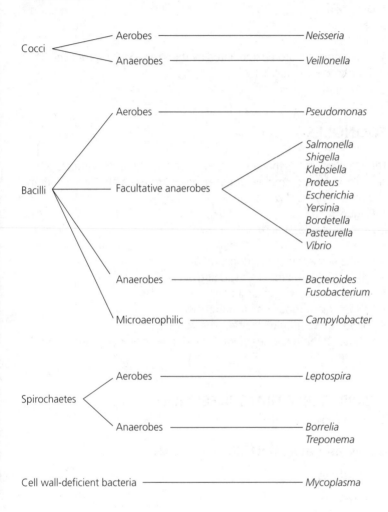

DISEASES CAUSED BY TOXINS

1 Diphtheria
2 Tetanus
3 Botulism
4 Toxic shock syndrome (mediated by the toxin TSST-1, produced by *Staphylococcus aureus*).

ZOONOSES

These are infections that are caused by an agent that also infects other animals or, less commonly, diseases which are spread between humans and other animals. Example include:
1 Plague (rats)
2 Anthrax (cattle, sheep)
3 Tularaemia (squirrels, rodents)
4 Leptospirosis (rats, pigs, dogs, cattle)
5 Lyme disease (mammals, including deer)
6 Brucellosis (cattle, goats, sheep)
7 Leishmaniasis (dogs, small mammals)
8 Salmonellosis (poultry, cattle, pigs, rodents)
9 Listeriosis (many species of wild and domestic animals, birds and fish).

RESPIRATORY TRACT INFECTIONS
(see also pages 378–381)

Upper respiratory tract infections (URTI)

Viral causes

1 Rhinoviruses
2 Coronaviruses
3 Adenoviruses
4 Parainfluenza viruses
5 Coxsackieviruses groups A and B
6 Respiratory syncytial virus.

Bacterial causes

1 Group A β-haemolytic streptococcus, *Steptococcus pyogenes*
2 *Haemophilus influenzae*
3 *Neisseria meningitidis* and *Neisseria gonorrhoeae* (mostly asymptomatic)
4 *Moraxella catarrhalis*
5 *Mycoplasma pneumoniae.*

Lower respiratory tract infections (LRTI)

Common causes

1 *Streptococcus pneumoniae*
2 *Haemophilus influenzae*
3 *Streptococcus pyogenes*
4 *Legionella pneumophila*
5 *Staphylococcus aureus*
6 *Mycoplasma pneumoniae*
7 *Klebsiella pneumoniae.*

Uncommon causes

1 *Chlamydia* spp.
2 *Coxiella burnetii*
3 *Leptospira icterohaemorrhagiae*
4 *Fusobacterium necrophorum*
5 *Salmonella typhi*
6 *Francisella tularensis*
7 *Yersinia pestis.*

Causes in immunocompromised patients

1 Pseudomonas spp.
2 *Pneumocystis*
3 *Aspergillus*
4 CMV.

Viral causes

1 RSV
2 Influenza virus
3 Parainfluenza virus.

GASTROINTESTINAL INFECTIONS (see also page 139)

1 Most gut infections cause diarrhoea
2 Small bowel infections are often toxin-mediated, with watery diarrhoea, usually non-bloody
3 Large bowel infections (with some exceptions) invade the colonic mucosa and cause bloody diarrhoea with mucus and sometimes pus – 'dysentery'.

Organisms that cause toxin-mediated infections of the small bowel

1 *Salmonella* spp. – from eggs and chickens (incubation period 12–48 hours)
2 Some *Campylobacter* species – account for most acute gastroenteritis in the UK (incubation 2–5 days)
3 Enterotoxigenic *E. coli* (ETEC) – main cause of traveller's diarrhoea (incubation 12–72 hours)
4 Rotavirus (incubation 1–7 days)
5 *Staphylcoccus aureus* (incubation 2–6 hours)
6 *Clostridium perfringens* (incubation 8–22 hours)
7 *Clostridium botulinium* – canned or bottled food (18–36 hours)
8 *Vibrio cholerae*
9 *Bacillus cereus/subtilis* – contaminated rice (incubation 1–5 hours emetic; 12–24 hours diarrhoeal)
10 *Yersinia enterocolitica* (incubation 24–36 hours)
11 *Giardia lamblia* (incubation 1–4 weeks)
12 *Aeromonas* spp.
13 Small round structured viruses.

Organisms that cause invasive infections of the large bowel

1 *Campylobacter* spp.
2 *Shigella* spp. (incubation 2–3 days)
3 *Yersinia enterocolitica*
4 Enteroinvasive *E. coli* (EIEC)
5 *Entamoeba histolytica* – presents similarly to ulcerative colitis but note that steroids can be lethal in amoebiasis.

Organisms that cause toxin-mediated infections of the large bowel

1 *Clostridium difficile*
2 Enterohaemorrhagic *E. coli* (EHEC) – typically serotype 0157, responsible for an epidemic form of haemolytic-uraemic syndrome, e.g. the Lanarkshire outbreak, 1999.

Hepatitis B

Serological markers

1 Hepatitis B surface antigen (*HBsAg*) – active infection with hepatitis B, acute or chronic
2 Hepatitis B 'e' antigen (*HBeAg*) – acute infection with hepatitis B or chronic carrier state of high infectivity
3 Antibodies to HBeAg (*anti-HBe*) – resolving acute infection with hepatitis B or a chronic carrier state of low infectivity
4 IgM antibodies to heptitis B core antigen (*anti-HBc-IgM*) – acute infection with hepatitis B
5 Total antibodies to hepatitis B core antigen (*anti-HBc*) – natural infection with hepatitis B at some time
6 Antibodies to HBsAg (*anti-HBs*) – immunity to hepatitis B, vaccine-induced or natural.

[See Table 33, overleaf]

URINARY TRACT INFECTIONS

Causative organisms

1 *Escherichia coli* – (most commonly serotypes O2, O4, O6, O7, O18, O75). Account for 60–90% UTIs
2 *Proteus mirabilis* – cause 10% UTIs
3 *Staphylococcus saprophyticus* – an important cause in sexually active women
4 *Klebsiella* spp.
5 *Streptococcus faecalis*
6 'Fastidious' Gram-postive bacteria, e.g. *Lactobacillus*, streptococci, corynebacteria

Table 33

	HBsAg	HBeAg	Anti-HBe	Anti-HBc-IgM	Anti-HBc (total)	Anti-HBs
Active infection with hepatitis B	+	+	–	+	+	–
Chronic carrier of high infectivity	+	+	–	–	+	–
Chronic carrier of intermediate infectivity	+	–	–	–	+	–
Chronic carrier of low infectivity	+	–	+	–	+	–
Infection with hepatitis B sometime in the past	–	–	±	–	+	–
Natural immunity to hepatitis B	–	–	±	–	+	+
Vaccine-induced immunity to hepatitis B	–	–	–	–	–	+

7 Opportunistic organisms after catheterisation, e.g. *Pseudomonas aeruginosa*, *Staphylococcus aureus*
8 *Mycobacterium tuberculosis*.

Suitable oral antibiotics

These are all excreted in urine:
1 Trimethoprim
2 Co-trimoxazole
3 Ampicillin
4 Co-amoxiclav
5 Nitrofurantoin
6 Nalidixic acid
7 Cefalexin.

SEXUALLY TRANSMITTED INFECTIONS

Gonorrhoea

1 Caused by infection with *Neisseria gonorrhoeae*
2 Transmission through oral, vaginal or anal intercourse
3 A large proportion are asymptomatic
4 Symptoms include pus-like urethral discharge, itch, pain
5 Sensitive to penicillin, ciprofloxacin, cephalosporin and tetracycline (UK)
6 Left untreated, leads to urethral strictures, pelvic inflammatory disease in women, prostatitis/epididymitis in men
7 Responsible for ophthalmia neonatorum.

Chlamydial infection

1 Caused by *Chlamydia trachomatis*
2 Responsible for over half of cases of non-specific urethritis (NSU), previously known as 'non-gonococcal urethritis' (NGU)
3 A cause of pelvic inflammatory disease and infertility in women
4 May cause conjunctivitis and a diffuse pneumonia in neonates
5 Sensitive to doxycycline and erythromycin.

Trichomoniasis

1 Caused by *Trichomonas vaginalis*, a flagellated protozoan

2 Causes foul-smelling, greeny/yellow vaginal discharge and vaginitis
3 Treated with metronidazole.

Herpes simplex

1 Caused by herpes simplex virus (HSV) types 1 and 2
2 Infection may remain dormant for very long periods
3 Causes painful genital ulceration
4 Aciclovir helps reduce duration of lesions
5 Can recur after the initial infection (but usually less aggressively).

Anogenital warts

1 Caused by human papilloma virus (HPV) – there are up to 60 different types
2 Benign tumours of the skin
3 Can cause large lesions around the anus, glans, labia or vagina, involving both skin and mucous membranes
4 Treated with cryotherapy and podophyllin
5 Often recur
6 Types 16 and 18 are associated with carcinoma of the cervix.

Syphilis

1 Caused by the spirochaete *Treponema pallidum*
2 Transmission mainly sexual; incubation 2–4 weeks
3 *Primary syphilis* – painless genital ulceration, the classical chancre. Heals in 3–8 weeks
4 *Secondary syphilis* – six to eight weeks later the infection becomes generalised with a rash, often papular. Generalised lymphadenopathy. Rare manifestations include periostitis, arthritis, hepatitis, glomerulonephritis
5 *Tertiary syphilis* – three to ten years after the primary lesion. Gummas (granulomatous nodules) form in skin, mucous membranes or bones. Gummas can break down to form shallow punched-out ulcers
6 *Late or quaternary syphilis* – ten to twenty years after primary syphilis. There are two main forms:
   (a) cardiovascular – aortitis, aneurysm, aortic incompetence, coronary ostial stenosis

(b) neurological:
  (i) tabes dorsalis (ataxic gait, trophic changes in joints (Charcot's), optic atrophy)
  (ii) general paralysis of the insane (dementia, tremor, spastic paralysis)
  (iii) meningovascular syphilis (headache, cranial nerve palsies, loss of papillary reaction to light (Argyll Robertson pupils)
7 Diagnosis is by direct demonstration of the spirochaete in fluid from a chancre or from an ulcerated secondary lesion
8 Treated with penicillin.

Serological tests for syphilis

The three main tests are:
1 The Venereal Disease Reference Laboratory (VDRL) test, a cardiolipin antibody test
2 The *Treponema pallidum* haemagglutination assay (TPHA) – a treponemal antibody test
3 The fluorescent treponemal antibody absorbed (FTA-Abs) test.

Table 34

Stage of disease	VDRL	TPHA	FTA-Abs
Primary	±	−	+
Late primary	+	±	+
Secondary and tertiary	+	+	+
Latent	+	+	+
Late	+	+	+
Treated	−	+	+
Congenital syphilis	+	+	+

NEUROLOGICAL INFECTIONS

Causes of meningitis

1 Acute bacterial:
  (a) adults:
    (i) meningococcus
    (ii) pneumococcus

   (b) neonates:
      (i) group B *Streptococcus*
      (ii) *E. coli*
   (c) Rarities – lymphocytic CSF:
      (i) *Listeria monocytogenes*
      (ii) leptospirosis
      (iii) syphilis
      (iv) Lyme disease
   (d) Rarities – polymorphs in CSF:
      (i) *Mycobacterium tuberculosis*
      (ii) *S. aureus*
2 Chronic bacterial: *Mycobacterium tuberculosis*
3 Chronic fungal: cryptococcosis
4 Acute viral:
   (a) mumps
   (b) enteroviruses (especially polio)
   (c) HSV
5 Miscellaneous:
   (a) cysticercial meningitis (*Taenia solium* and *Taenia saginata*)
   (b) amoebic meningitis.

Causes of encephalitis (see also pages 308–309)

1 Viral causes:
   (a) herpes simplex (mainly type 1)
   (b) enteroviruses
   (c) arboviruses (e.g. Japanese encephalitis)
   (d) varicella zoster
   (e) HIV
   (f) rabies
2 Toxoplasmosis
3 Cysticercosis (pig/bovine tapeworms)
4 African trypanosomiasis ('sleeping sickness' – *Trypanosoma brucei rhodesiense*).

Cerebrospinal fluid (see also pages 334–336)

[See Table 35, opposite]

Table 35

	Normal CSF	Acute bacterial meningitis	Acute viral meningitis	*Mycobacterium tuberculosis* infection	Multiple sclerosis
Appearance	Crystal clear, colourless	Turbid/purulent	Clear/turbid	Turbid/viscous	Normal
Glucose level	Two-thirds to one-half of blood glucose level	Low	Normal or high	Low	Normal
Protein level	0.2–0.4 g/litre	Very high	High	Very high	High
Mononuclear cell count	5/mm^3	< 50/mm^3	10–100/mm^3	100–300/mm^3	5–60/mm^3
Polymorph cell count	Nil	200–3000/mm^3	Nil (early rise)	0–200/mm^3	—
Microbiology	Nil	Gram-stain and blood culture etc.	Throat swab and serology etc.	AAFB on ZN staining	IgG >15% of normal Oligoclonal band positive
Pressure	60–150mm of H$_2$O with patient lying down	Normal or raised	Normal or raised	Normal or raised	Normal or raised

HELMINTH INFECTIONS

Cestode (tapeworm) infections

1 *Taenia saginata* (beef)
2 *Taenia solium* (pork) – may lead to cysticercosis
3 *Diphyllobothrium latum* (fish)
4 *Echinococcus granulosus* (dogs) – causes cystic hydatid disease.

Nematode (roundworm) infections

1 *Necator americanus* and *Ancylostoma duodenale* (hookworms). Larvae penetrate the feet. Leads to iron deficiency anaemia
2 *Strongyloides stercoralis* – may cause malabsorption
3 *Ascaris lumbricoides* – looks like an earthworm. Can cause GI obstruction
4 *Trichinella spiralis* – transmitted by uncooked pork. Migrates to muscle
5 *Enterobius vermicularis* – (threadworm/pinworm). Causes pruritus ani. Commonest helmintic infection in the UK
6 *Toxicara canis* or *T. cati* (dog/cat roundworms). Cause visceral larva migricans (toxocariasis)
7 *Ancylostoma braziliense* and *A. cannum* (non-human hookworms). Cause cutaneous larva migricans
8 *Dracunculus medinensis* (Guinea worm) – a very long worm which emerges through the skin
9 Filariasis (very common):
    (a) *Onchocerca volvulus* – causes blindness
    (b) *Wuchereria bancrofti* and *Brugia malayi* – cause lymphangitis, elephantiasis and tropical pulmonary eosinophilia
    (c) *Loa loa* – may migrate through subconjunctival tissue.

Trematode (fluke) infections

1 Schistosomiasis (bilharzia) – caused by *Schistosoma haematobium* (inferior pelvic veins), and *S. mansoni* and *S. japonicum* (mesenteric veins)
2 *Fasciola hepatica* (liver fluke)
3 *Paragonimus westermani* (lung fluke).

TROPICAL INFECTIOUS DISEASES

[See Table 36, overleaf]

PROTOZOAL INFECTIONS

Intestinal

1 *Cryptosporidium parvum*
2 *Giardia lamblia*
3 *Entamoeba histolytica.*

Blood and tissue

1 Malaria
2 Leishmaniasis
3 Trypanosomiasis
4 Toxoplasmosis (serological tests required)
5 Babeosis.

RICKETTSIAL INFECTIONS

1 Micro-organisms that are usually classified as bacteria but which demonstrate some characteristics of viruses
2 Cause typhus and spotted fevers
3 Transmitted by arthropod vectors
4 Incubation period one to two weeks
5 Cause an acute febrile illness with rash, headache, malaise and haemorrhage
6 Rash is maculopapular. Petechiae are common in spotted fevers
7 An eschar (a skin ulcer with a blackened centre) may be seen at the site of the tick bite
8 Fatality varies: in untreated typhus it may be as high as 10–15%; in untreated Rocky Mountain fever ranges from 15% to 20%
9 Treated with tetracycline chloramphenicol or ciprofloxacin.

[See Table 37, page 251]

Table 36

Disease	Parasite	Vector
Schistosomiasis (bilharzia)	*Schistosoma mansoni, S. japonicum, S. haematobium*	Freshwater snails
Guinea worm	*Dracunculus medinensis*	Cyclops (water flea)
Onchocerciasis (blinding worm)	*Onchocerca volvulus*	*Simulium damnosum* (buffalo fly)
Loiasis (eye worm)	*Loa loa*	*Chrysops* flies
Paragonimiasis (lung fluke)	*Paragonimus westermani*	Crustaceans
Leishmaniasis:		
Visceral leishmaniasis (kala-azar)	*Leishmania donovani, L. infantum*	Sandflies
Cutaneous leishmaiasis	*L. tropica, L. major*	
Mucocutaneous leishmaniasis (including espundia)	*L. braziliensis*	
	Trypanosoma, L. mexicana	
African trypanosomiasis – (sleeping sickness)	*Trypanosoma brucei rhodesiense, T. brucei gambiense*	Tsetse flies
South American trypanosomiasis (Chagas' disease)	*T. cruzi*	Riduvid insects
Malaria	*Plasmodium falciparum, P. vivax, P. ovale, P. malariae*	Mosquitoes

Table 37

Disease	Organism	Reservoir	Vector	Geographical distribution
Typhus group				
Epidemic typhus	*Rickettsia prowazeki*	Man	Louse	America, Africa, Asia
Murine typhus	*R. typhi*	Rats, mice	Fleas	Worldwide
Scrub typhus	*R. tsutsugamushi*	Rodents	Mites	Far East
Spotted fever group				
Rocky Mountain spotted fever	*R. rickettsii*	Rodents, dogs	Ticks	North and South America
Boutonneuse fever	*R. conori*	Rodents, dogs	Ticks	Mediterranean, Africa, India
Queensland tick typhus	*R. australis*	Rodents, marsupials	Ticks	Australia
North Asian tick fever	*R. siberica*	Ticks, ?rodents, ?hares	Ticks	Eastern Russia, China, Mongolia
Rickettsial pox	*R. akari*	House mice	Mites	USA, Russia

FUNGAL INFECTIONS

1 Aerobic organisms
2 Readily grown on simple media
3 Ubiquitous in nature
4 Often pose a problem in immunocompromised patients
5 Can be grouped into three major categories:
   (a) yeasts
   (b) filamentous fungi
   (c) dimorphic fungi.

Yeasts

1 *Candida albicans* – infects mucous membranes (thrush); may cause chronic mucocutaneous candidiasis; can involve lower respiratory and urinary tracts, eye, meninges, kidney and bone
2 *Cryptococcus neoformans* – a lung granuloma is normally the primary focus, subsequent haematogenous spread leading to subacute or chronic meningoencephalitis.

Filamentous fungi

1 Dermatophytes – *Tinea* (ringworm). Affects nails, skin, hair
2 *Aspergillus* spp. – can cause a variety of clinical syndromes: allergic bronchopulmonary aspergillosis (ABPA), aspergilloma, invasive aspergillosis, superficial infections
3 Zymomycosis may be caused by *Mucor, Rhizopus, Absidia* and *Conidiobolus* fungi
4 *Penicilium* spp.

Dimorphic fungi

1 *Coccidioides immitis*
2 *Histoplasma capsulatum*
3 *Blastomyces dermatitidis.*

Metabolic Medicine

LIPIDS

Lipoproteins

1 *Very low density lipoprotein (VLDL):*
   (a) synthesised continuously by liver
   (b) carries 60% triglycerides and some cholesterol
   (c) enzymic degradation to intermediate density lipoprotein (IDL) and
       then LDL
2 *Low density lipoprotein (LDL):*
   (a) formed from IDL by hepatic lipase
   (b) major carrier of cholesterol
   (c) binds to, and levels regulated by feedback onto hepatic LDL
       receptor
3 *High density lipoprotein (HDL):*
   (a) synthesised in gut wall and liver
   (b) carries cholesterol from periphery to liver
   (c) inverse association with ischaemic heart disease
4 *Chylomicrons:*
   (a) carry dietary lipid from gut to liver
   (b) broken down by lipoprotein lipase in portal vessels to free fatty
       acids.

Hyperlipidaemias

1 Can be primary or secondary
2 Atherosclerotic disease associated with high total cholesterol and LDL
3 HDL is protective.

Primary disorders

Familial hypercholesterolaemia

1 Autosomal dominant; heterozygotes 1 in 500 of normal population
2 Over 400 defects in LDL receptor known
3 Total cholesterol 9–15 mmol/l
4 Six to eight times increased risk of IHD (MI at young age)
5 Other features are xanthelasma and tendon xanthomata
6 Treat with diet and statins.

Familial triglyceridaemia

1 Autosomal dominant
2 Plasma turbid
3 Associated with eruptive xanthomata, pancreatitis, retinal vein thrombosis, hepatosplenomegaly, lipaemia retinalis
4 Treat with diet and fibrates.

Lipoprotein lipase deficiency

1 Rare
2 Failure to break down chylomicrons.

Familial combined hyperlipidaemia

1 Elevated cholesterol and triglycerides
2 Prevalence 1:200
3 Main feature is atherosclerosis.

Causes of secondary hyperlipidaemia

1 Mainly raised cholesterol:
   (a) hypothyroidism
   (b) cholestasis
   (c) nephrotic syndrome
   (d) renal transplant
2 Mainly raised triglycerides:
   (a) obesity
   (b) chronic alcohol excess
   (c) insulin resistance and diabetes
   (d) chronic liver disease

(e) thiazide diuretics
(f) high-dose oestrogens.

BONE AND MINERALS

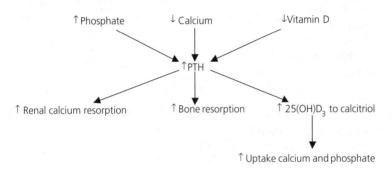

Vitamin D

1 Mostly made in skin by action of UV light
2 25-hydroxylated in the liver
3 Hydroxylated again to $1,25(OH)_2D_3$ (calcitriol) in the kidney.

Hypercalcaemia

Causes

1 Primary hyperparathyroidism (adenoma of parathyroid gland)
2 Malignancy (bone metastases plus PTH-related protein), commonly breast, kidney or squamous cell tumours
3 ↑ Calcium intake (and milk-alkali syndrome)
4 ↑ Vitamin D
5 Tertiary hyperparathyroidism
6 Hyperthyroidism
7 Sarcoid (macrophages in lesions produce $1,25 D_3$)
8 Thiazides
9 Lithium
10 Addison's disease
11 Theophylline toxicity
12 Phaeochromocytoma
13 Familial hypocalciuric hypercalcaemia.

Features

1 As underlying condition, plus
2 Lethargy, malaise and depression
3 Weakness
4 Confusion
5 Constipation
6 Nausea
7 Renal stones
8 Diabetes insipidus
9 Pancreatitis.

Treatment

1 Aggressive rehydration
2 Intravenous diphosphonate (pamidronate).

Hyperparathyroidism

1 *Primary:*
   (a) single adenoma in >80%
   (b) multiple in around 5%
   (c) commonest in women aged 40–60 years
   (d) carcinoma very rare
   (e) results in ↑ PTH, ↑ serum and urinary calcium,↑ ALP and ↓ serum phosphate
   (f) causes increased osteoblasts and osteoclasts and therefore own turnover (bone loss can occur)
2 *Secondary:* Due to hypertrophy of glands in response to chronic hypocalcaemia (e.g. in renal failure)
3 *Tertiary:* Consequence of long-standing secondary hyperparathyroidism. Further gland hyperplasia raises calcium levels. Treatment is parathyroidectomy.

Hypocalcaemia

Causes

1 Hypoparathyroidism
2 Low levels of vitamin D_3
3 Hyperphosphataemia
4 Hypomagnesaemia

5 Sepsis
6 Respiratory alkalosis
7 Calcium deposition (pancreatitis).

Features

1 Muscle weakness
2 Neuromuscular excitability
3 Confusion seizures
4 Tetany
5 Alopecia
6 Brittle nails
7 Cataracts
8 Dental hypoplasia.

Treatment

Supplementation of calcium, vitamin D_3.

Causes of hypoparathyroidism

1 Parathyroidectomy (intentional or accidental)
2 Autoimmune
3 Receptor defect (pseudo-hyperparathyroidism).

Causes of hyperphosphataemia

1 Renal failure
2 Hypoparathyroidism
3 Acromegaly
4 Vitamin D excess
5 Over-intake of phosphate
6 Tumour lysis syndrome.

Causes of hypophosphataemia

1 Intravenous glucose
2 Total parenteral nutrition
3 Recovery phase of diabetic ketoacidosis
4 Primary hyperparathyroidism
5 Renal tubular disease

6 Vitamin D deficiency.

Osteomalacia/rickets

Decreased mineralisation of osteoid.

Causes

1 Calciopenic:
   (a) vitamin D deficiency
   (b) impaired calcium metabolism
2 Phosphopenic: proximal renal tubular disease.

Clinical features

1 Pain
2 Deformity
3 Fractures
4 Proximal myopathy
5 Raised ALP.

Paget's disease

1 Increased bone turnover with abnormal new bone turnover
2 Causes pain, deformity, arthritis, nerve compression, fractures, sarcoma
3 Associated with greatly raised ALP; calcium only raised with immobility
4 Treatment mainly analgesia. Can use bisphosphonates.

Osteoporosis (see also page 413)

1 Reduced bone mass and density
2 Abnormal bone microarchitecture
3 May be primary or secondary.

Primary

1 *Type I:* oestrogen deficiency post-menopause. Affects mainly trabecular bone
2 *Type II:* age-related decrease in osteoblastic activity. Affects cortical and trabecular bone.

Secondary

1 Drugs:
   (a) steroids
   (b) heparin
   (c) antiepileptics
   (d) ciclosporin A
2 Endocrine:
   (a) Cushing's syndrome
   (b) hyperparathyroidism
   (c) prolactinoma
   (d) premature menopause
   (e) hyperthyroidism
   (f) hypogonadism
3 Malignancy:
   (a) myeloma
   (b) leukaemia
4 GI:
   (a) malabsorption syndromes
   (b) post-gastrectomy
   (c) PBC
5 Inflammatory disorders:
   (a) ulcerative colitis
   (b) RA
6 Immobilisation:
   (a) non-weight-bearing (space flight)
7 Other causes:
   (a) alcoholism
   (b) osteogenesis imperfecta
   (c) Turner's syndrome.

Tests

1 Calcium, phosphate, ALP normal
2 Diagnosis by DEXA scan
3 Markers of bone resorption:
   (a) collagen cross-linking telepeptides
   (b) pyridinium cross-links
4 Markers of bone formation:
   (a) osteocalcin

(b)   pro-collagen terminal peptides.

Treatment

1 Treatment of any secondary cause
2 HRT
3 Calcium and vitamin D
4 Calcitonin
5 Bisphosphonates.

MAGNESIUM

Hypomagnesaemia

1 Usually associated with low calcium and low potassium
2 Associated with ventricular arrhythmias.

Causes

1 *Renal loss:*
    (a)   loop/thiazide diuretics
    (b)   alcohol
    (c)   diabetic ketoacidasis
    (d)   volume expansion
    (e)   hypercalcaemia
2 *Loop of Henle disorder:*
    (a)   acute tubular necrosis
    (b)   post-obstruction diuresis
    (c)   renal transplant
3 *Nephrotoxic drugs:*
    (a)   aminoglycosides
    (b)   cisplatin
    (c)   ciclosporin A
    (d)   amphotericin B
    (e)   pentamidine
4 *GI loss:*
    (a)   high-volume diarrhoea
    (b)   malabsorption
    (c)   other small bowel disease
    (d)   acute pancreatitis

5 *Primary renal magnesium wasting:* a rare familial condition.

Hypermagnesaemia

Causes

1 Magnesium infusion
2 Magnesium enema
3 Oral magnesium overdose
4 Renal failure
5 Adrenal insufficiency
6 Milk-alkali syndrome
7 Theophylline toxicity
8 Lithium.

Treat with intravenous calcium if symptomatic.

COPPER

1 Half of ingested copper is absorbed
2 Transported to the liver by albumin
3 Binds with globulin to form caeruloplasmin.

Wilson's disease

1 Autosomal recessive
2 Gene on chromosome 3
3 Abnormality of caeruloplasmin formation leading to accumulation of copper in the body
4 *Features:*
   (a) acute/chronic hepatitis
   (b) cirrhosis
   (c) Kayser-Fleischer rings
   (d) CNS symptoms
   (e) arthropathy
5 *Diagnosis:*
   (a) low caeruloplasmin
   (b) high urinary copper
   (c) liver biopsy
6 *Treatment:*
   (a) penicillamine (copper chelator)

(b) liver transplant.

IRON

1 The normal human body contains 4 g iron; haemoglobin 2–3 g
2 Normal diet contains 20 mg per day; only 10% absorbed
3 Fe^{2+} more readily absorbed than Fe^{3+}
4 Transferrin normally one-third saturated
5 Ferritin (acute phase protein) increased in iron overload, decreased in deficiency
6 Plasma iron varies greatly.

Haemochromatosis

1 Autosomal recessive
2 More common and more severe in men
3 Gene on chromosome 6
4 *Features:*
    (a) micronodular cirrhosis
    (b) chondrocalcinosis
    (c) pseudogout
    (d) skin bronzing
    (e) diabetes
    (f) cardiomyopathy
    (g) arrhythmias
5 *Diagnosis:*
    (a) raised serum iron and ferritin, transferrin >60% saturated
    (b) HFE gene testing
    (c) liver biopsy
6 *Treatment:*
    (a) venesection
    (b) desferrioxamine.

Causes of secondary iron overload

1 Multiple transfusions
2 Alcoholic cirrhosis
3 Chronic hepatitis B/C
4 Beta-thalassaemia

5 Aplastic anaemia
6 Sideroblastic anaemia.

PORPHYRIAS (see also page 53)

1 Hereditary defects of enzymes involved in the haem synthesis pathway
2 Overproduction of intermediates (porphyrins)
3 Several different types. Most important are acute intermittent porphyria and porphyria cutanea tarda.

Acute intermittent porphyria

1 Autosomal dominant
2 Rare, more common in females
3 Due to low levels of porphobilinogen deaminase in the liver
4 Presents in youth
5 Increased urinary porphobilinogen in attacks: urine turns dark red after standing
6 *Features:*
   (a) abdominal pain
   (b) neuropsychiatric symptoms
   (c) vomiting
   (d) hypertension
   (e) tachycardia
   (f) motor polyneuropathy
7 Commonly precipitated by hepatic enzyme-inducing drugs, e.g. alcohol, phenytoin, oral contraceptives, sulphonamides, rifampicin, benzodiazepines.

Porphyria cutanea tarda

1 Chronic hepatic condition
2 Probably autosomal dominant
3 Accumulation of uroporphyrinogen (urine levels raised)
4 Photosensitive rash is the main feature.

AMINO ACID METABOLISM DISORDERS

[See Table 38, overleaf]

Table 38

Condition	Genetics	Clinical features	Diagnosis	Management
Cystinosis	AR (short arm of 17)	Lymhadenopathy Growth retardation Fanconi syndrome Renal failure	Measure cystine content of neutrophils	Dialysis Renal transplant Usually fatal
Cystinuria	AR	Renal stones	Urinary cystine/stone analysis	Fluids Penicillamine Alkalisation of urine
Homocystinuria	AR	Osteoporosis Arterial thrombosis Downward dislocation of lens Mental retardation	Cyanide-nitroprusside test – raised urinary homocysteine	Methionine restriction Supplements of cystine and pyridoxine
Alkaptonuria	AR	Arthritis Disc calcification Pigmentation of ears	Clinical features Urine darkens on standing	Symptomatic, for arthritis
Phenylketonuria	AR	Mental retardation Irritability Eczema Decreased pigmentation	Guthrie screening test perinatally	Dietary restriction of phenylalanine Tyrosine supplements
Oxalosis	AR	Renal stones/calcification Bone, cardiac and arterial disease	Urinary oxalate increased May need liver biopsy	Pyridoxine Treat renal failure Fluids ?? Liver transplant

DEFICIENCIES

Protein–energy malnutrition

1 *Undernutrition:* weight 60–80% of standard for age, no oedema
2 *Marasmus:*
   (a) deficient in protein and calories
   (b) weight <60% of standard, no oedema
3 *Kwashiorkor:*
   (a) solely due to protein deficiency
   (b) weight 60–80% of standard, oedema present
   (c) fatty liver often seen.

Vitamin deficiencies

Table 39

Vitamin	Cause of deficiency	Consequence of deficiency
A	Protein–energy malnutrition	Night blindness Dry cornea Keratomalacia
B_1 (thiamine)	Alcoholism Dietary restriction	Dry beriberi: Wernicke–Korsakoff polyneuropathy Wet beriberi: high-output cardiac failure
B_2 (riboflavin)	Protein–energy malnutrition	Glossitis Angular stomatitis
Niacin	Alcoholism Isoniazid Carcinoid syndrome	Pellagra – **d**ermatitis, **d**iarrhoea, **d**ementia and **d**eath
B_6 (pyridoxine)	Hydralazine Isoniazid	Peripheral neuropathy Glossitis
B_{12} (cyanocobalamin)	Pernicious anaemia Gastrectomy Ileal disease Vegans	Macrocytic anaemia Subacute combined degeneration of the cord
C	Dietary deficiency	Scurvy: gingivitis, bleeding, joint swelling
D	Renal failure Dietary	Osteomalacia/rickets
E	Fat malabsorption Abetalipoproteinaemia	Spinocerebellar degeneration
K	Biliary obstruction Antibiotic therapy	Bleeding diathesis

Nephrology

PHYSIOLOGY

Glomerular filtration rate (GFR)

1 Passive process
2 Normal values/corrected to height 1.73 m: 130 ml/minute in males; 120 ml/minute in females
3 Calculating GFR:
   (a) 24-hour urine collection
   (b) Cockcroft and Gault equation:

$$GFR = \frac{(140 - age\ in\ years) \times weight\ (kg)}{serum\ creatinine\ (\mu mol/l)} \times 1.23\ (male)\ or\ 1.04\ (female)$$

   (c) inulin clearance
   (d) radioisotope studies.

The renal tubule

Proximal tubule

1 50% sodium reabsorbed
2 90% bicarbonate reabsorbed
3 Phosphate reabsorption (PTH -dependent)
4 Drug secretion into urine – trimethoprim, cimetidine, most diuretics
5 Creatinine and urate secretion.

Loop of Henle

1 Medullary concentration gradient
2 40% sodium reabsorption
3 Loop diuretic action, e.g. furosemide (frusemide).

Distal tubule

1 5% sodium reabsorption
2 Thiazide diuretic action
3 Aldosterone receptors.

Collecting duct

1 2% sodium reabsorption
2 Spironolactone acts on aldosterone receptors
3 Hydrogen ion secretion (acidifying urine)
4 Antidiuretic hormone action.

Urea and creatinine

Causes of raised creatinine

1 Large muscle bulk
2 Rhabdomyolysis
3 Decreased tubular secretion, e.g. trimethoprim, potassium-sparing diuretics.

Causes of reduced creatinine

1 Small muscle mass
2 Pregnancy
3 Raised ADH.

Causes of raised urea

1 Reduced GFR, e.g. dehydration
2 GI bleeding
3 Corticosteroids/tetracycline
4 High protein diet
5 Increased catabolism.

Causes of reduced urea

1 Liver disease, e.g. excess alcohol
2 Starvation/anabolic state
3 Raised ADH
4 Pregnancy.

Causes of coloured urine

1 Haematuria
2 Haemoglobinuria
3 Drugs, e.g. rifampicin
4 Beetroot
5 Myoglobinuria
6 Obstructive jaundice
7 Porphyria
8 Alkaptonuria.

Renal tubular acidosis (RTA)

Table 40

	Type 1 (Distal)	Type 2 (Proximal)
Defect	Impaired acidification of urine	Defect in reabsorption of bicarbonate
Urine pH	>5.3 (never acidified)	Can vary
Plasma bicarbonate	<10 mmol/l	14–20 mmol/l
Plasma K	Low	Normal or low
Complications	Nephrocalcinosis	Osteomalacia (excretion of phosphate)
	Calculi	Rickets
	Growth failure	Fanconi syndrome
	UTIs	
Diagnosis	Ammonium chloride load fails to acidify urine	Fractional bicarbonate rises after i.v. bicarbonate load

Causes of type 1 RTA

1 SLE
2 Sjögren's syndrome
3 Chronic active hepatitis
4 Chronic pyelonephritis
5 Chronic interstitial nephritis
6 Obstructive nephropathy
7 Rejection in transplant
8 Medullary sponge kidney
9 Hypercalcaemia

10 Lithium
11 Amphotericin
12 Toluene
13 Idiopathic.

Causes of type 2 RTA

 1 Wilson's disease
 2 Cystinosis
 3 Sjögren's syndrome
 4 Fructose intolerance
 5 Interstitial nephritis
 6 Amyloidosis
 7 Tetracycline (past sell-by date)
 8 Myeloma
 9 Sulphonamides
10 Acetazolamide
11 Lead
12 Mercury.

Causes of type 4 RTA

1 Hyperkalaemia
2 Mild renal impairment
3 Hyporeninaemic hypoaldosteronism
4 Can occur in association with:
   (a) diabetic nephropathy
   (b) hypoadrenalism
   (c) gout nephropathy
   (d) urinary obstruction
   (e) NSAIDs
   (f) potassium-sparing diuretics.

ACUTE RENAL FAILURE

Causes

1 Prerenal: appropriate renal response to poor renal perfusion
2 Renal:

(a) acute tubular necrosis:
    (i) following circulatory compromise
    (ii) following nephrotoxins (including toxins)
    (iii) commonly in sepsis
    (iv) often multiple causes
(b) vascular causes:
    (i) large vessel occlusion
    (ii) small vessel disease
    (iii) accelerated hypertension
    (iv) scleroderma
(c) glomerulonephritis
(d) interstitial nephritis
(e) vasculitis
(f) haematological:
    (i) myeloma
    (ii) haemolytic uraemic syndrome
(g) other causes:
    (i) rhabdomyolysis
    (ii) hepatorenal syndrome
    (iii) acute cortical necrosis
3 Postrenal: urinary obstruction.

Life-threatening conditions associated with ARF

Hyperkalaemia

Recognised by ECG changes as potassium increases:
1 Tenting of T waves
2 Reduction in size of P waves
3 Increase in PR interval
4 Widening QRS complexes
5 Disappearance of P waves
6 Further QRS widening
7 Sinusoidal waveform.

Treatment

1 Intravenous calcium (gluconate 10%, 10 ml over 60 seconds)
2 Intravenous insulin and dextrose
3 Calcium resonium
4 Furosemide (frusemide)

5 Salbutamol nebulisers
6 Dialysis.

Intravascular volume depletion

Demonstrated by low JVP, postural drop in blood pressure. Treated by rapid correction with intravenous blood, colloid or saline.

Investigation

1 *Full history and examination:*
   (a) ?systemic cause
   (b) drug history (penicillin or NSAIDs)
2 *Ultrasound scan:*
   (a) rule out obstruction
   (b) kidney size (if small renal failure is acute on chronic)
3 *Urine testing:*
   (a) microscopy of urine
   (b) stix and biochemical tests
4 *Intravenous urogram (IVU)*
5 *Isotope renography:*
   (a) static (e.g. DMSA)
   (b) dynamic (e.g. MAG3, DTPA)
   (c) captopril renogram to look for renovascular disease
6 *Specific blood tests:*
   (a) anti-GBM antibodies – Goodpasture's syndrome
   (b) ANCA – systemic vasculitis
   (c) anti-dsDNA and anti-Sm antibodies – systemic lupus erythematosus
   (d) C3 nephritic factor – mesangiocapillary glomerulonephritis (MCGN) type 2
   (e) ASOT and anti-DNAase – poststreptococcal glomerulonephritis
   (f) blood cultures – infection-related, especially endocarditis
7 *Non-specific blood tests:*
   (a) complement:
      (i) low in SLE, MCGN type 1 and type 2, mixed essential cryoglobulinaemia, post-infectious
      (ii) high in vasculitis
   (b) immunoglobulins:
      (i) polyclonal increase in SLE, vasculitis, post-infectious, sarcoid

(ii) monoclonal increase in myeloma
(iii) raised IgE in Churg–Strauss syndrome
(iv) raised IgA in Henoch–Schönlein purpura and IgA nephropathy
(c) cryoglobulins:
    (i) cryoglobulinaemia
    (ii) SLE and post-infectious
(d) CRP: increased in most cases but not usually in SLE
(e) neutrophilia, thrombocytosis: systemic vasculitis
(f) eosinophilia:
    (i) drug-induced interstitial nephritis
    (ii) Churg–Strauss syndrome
(g) lymphopenia: SLE
(h) thrombocytopenia:
    (i) drug-induced interstitial nephritis
    (ii) SLE.

Inflammatory conditions leading to ARF

1 *Acute glomerulonephritis:*
  (a) primary GN:
    (i) mesangial IgA nephropathy
    (ii) mesangiocapillary GN
  (b) infection-related GN:
    (i) post-infection (streptococcal)
    (ii) infective endocarditis
    (iii) ventricular shunt infection
    (iv) other infections, e.g. abscesses
2 *Acute interstitial nephritis:*
  (a) drug-related:
    (i) antibiotics (ampicillin, methicillin, rifampicin, sulphonamides)
    (ii) NSAIDs (fenoprofen, mefenamic acid)
    (iii) diuretics (thiazides, triamterene)
    (iv) others (e.g. allopurinol, cimetidine)
  (b) infection-related:
    (i) UTI
    (ii) *Legionella*
    (iii) Epstein–Barr virus
    (iv) leptospiral infection
    (v) hantavirus
3 *Systemic disease:*

(a) SLE
(b) sarcoidosis
4 *Malignancy*, especially myeloma
5 *Idiopathic*
6 *Vasculitis:*
   (a) Goodpasture's syndrome
   (b) primary systemic vasculitis:
      (i) Wegener's granulomatosis
      (ii) microscopic polyangiitis
      (iii) Churg–Strauss syndrome
      (iv) Henoch–Schonlein purpura.

Criteria for urgent renal replacement therapy

1 Severe hyperkalaemia
2 Fluid overload leading to pulmonary oedema
3 Acidosis resulting in circulatory compromise
4 Uraemia causing:
   (a) encephalopathy
   (b) pericarditis
   (c) bleeding.

Acute tubular necrosis (ATN)

1 Ischaemic damage
2 Renal hypoperfusion
3 Reversible in time but time taken varies (may need dialysis until recovery occurs).

It is important to distinguish between ATN and prerenal uraemia:
1 Prerenal uraemia produces low-volume, concentrated urine
2 ATN produces low- or high-volume, dilute, 'poor quality' urine.

Rhabdomyolysis

1 Muscle damage
2 Myoglobin release
3 ARF
4 Raised potassium and phosphate
5 Creatinine kinase massively raised
6 Creatinine raised disproportionately to urea.

Causes

1 Trauma/compression injury
2 Uncontrolled fitting
3 Statins
4 Burns
5 Infectious mononucleosis
6 Viral necrotising myositis
7 Barbiturate, alcohol or heroin overdose
8 Severe exercise
9 Heatstroke
10 Polymyositis
11 Malignant hyperpyrexia.

CHRONIC RENAL FAILURE

Causes (UK)

1 Diabetes mellitus (20%)
2 Chronic GN (20%)
3 Renovascular (15%)
4 Chronic reflux nephropathy (15%)
5 Polycystic kidney disease (10%)
6 Postobstructive (10%)
7 Myeloma (3%)
8 Amyloidosis (3%)
9 Other causes:
   (a) chronic interstitial nephritis
   (b) analgesic nephropathy
   (c) renal calculi
   (d) post-acute renal failure
   (e) other hereditary disorders.

Management of chronic renal disease

1 Blood pressure control:
   (a) ACE inhibitors
   (b) other hypertensives
   (c) diuretics
2 Reduction in proteinuria: ACE inhibitors

3 Treatment of anaemia:
   (a) intravenous iron
   (b) erythropoietin
4 Diet:
   (a) low salt intake
   (b) low potassium intake
   (c) high calorie intake
5 Treatment of hyperphosphataemia and hypocalcaemia:
   (a) phosphate binders
   (b) alphacalcidol
6 Glucose control in diabetics
7 Hyperlipidaemia control
8 Volume status monitoring and maintenance
9 Avoidance of nephrotoxic drugs
10 Awareness of risk of radiocontrast nephropathy.

Causes of hyperkalaemia

1 Spurious:
   (a) haemolysis
   (b) delayed separation of serum
   (c) contamination
2 Excessive intake:
   (a) oral (uncommon)
   (b) parenteral
3 Decreased excretion:
   (a) acute oliguric renal failure
   (b) chronic renal failure
   (c) potassium-sparing diuretics
   (d) ACE inhibitors
   (e) mineralocorticoid deficiency (Addison's disease)
4 Redistribution:
   (a) tissue damage
   (b) catabolic states
   (c) acidosis.

Causes of hypokalaemia

1 Decreased intake:
   (a) oral (uncommon, except in starvation)

(b) parental
2 Increased excretion:
   (a) gastrointestinal (e.g. diarrhoea, vomiting, drainage, fistulae, purgative abuse, villous adenoma)
   (b) renal (e.g. loop or thiazide diuretics, diuretic phase of ARF, mineralocorticoid excess, renal tubular acidosis)
3 Redistribution:
   (a) insulin, alkalosis
   (b) rapid cellular proliferation.

Long-term complications of dialysis

1 Anaemia
2 Vascular disease
3 Dialysis amyloid
4 Renal osteodystrophy
5 Acquired cystic disease
6 Aluminium toxicity (rare).

Anaemia of chronic renal failure

Anaemia occurs at GFR <35 ml/minute.

Causes

1 Lack of erythropoietin (normally produced by the kidneys) is the most important cause
2 Reduced iron intake
3 Impaired iron absorption
4 Toxic effect of uraemia on bone marrow
5 Capillary fragility
6 Reduced RBC survival.

Management

1 Subcutaneous erythropoietin (EPO) injections
2 Check ferritin/transferrin saturation
3 If ferritin <100 μg then give intravenous iron (Venofer®).

Causes of resistance to EPO therapy

1 Iron deficiency
2 Sepsis or chronic inflammation
3 GI blood loss
4 Hyperparathyroidism
5 Aluminium toxicity (now rare).

Renal osteodystrophy

Causative factors

1 Low plasma ionised calcium:
   (a) lack of 1,25 $(OH)_2$ vitamin D
   (b) malnutrition
   (c) hyperphosphataemia
2 Stimulation of parathyroid hormone release (secondary hyperparathyroidism) in response to:
   (a) hypocalcaemia
   (b) hyperphosphataemia
   (c) low 1,25 $(OH)_2$ vitamin D
3 Low vitamin D levels
4 Acidosis.

Treatment

1 Phosphate binders (e.g. calcium acetate) to lower phosphate levels
2 Bicarbonate
3 Vitamin D (1-alphacalcidol)
4 Parathyroidectomy may be necessary.

Haemodialysis *versus* peritoneal dialysis

Haemodialysis is favoured in the following conditions:
1 Recent abdominal surgery or irremediable hernia
2 Recurrent or persistent peritonitis (e.g. *Pseudomonas* or fungal infection)
3 Peritoneal membrane failure
4 Severe malnutrition – protein loss during dialysis
5 Intercurrent severe illness with hypercatabolism
6 Chronic severe respiratory disease
7 Age and general physical or mental frailty

8 Loss of residual renal function.

Renal transplantation

Two thousand patients per year undergo renal transplantation in the UK.
Graft survival is 90% at one year; 70% at five years.
Live donors account for 10–15% of transplants. *Contraindications to live
donation* include:
1 Pre-existing renal disease
2 Disease of unknown aetiology (e.g. MS or sarcoid)
3 Overt ischaemic heart disease.

Nephrectomy is carried out prior to transplant in the following
circumstances:
1 Uncontrollable hypertension
2 Infection in the urinary tract
3 Massive kidneys (e.g. polycystic disease)
4 Renal or urothelial malignancy (must be over two years
   recurrence-free prior to transplant).

HLA typing

1 Antigens on chromosome 6
2 Importance of HLA matching: DR > B > A > C
3 Acceptable: one DR or one B mismatch
4 Good match: no DR with no or one B mismatch.

Post-transplant complications

1 Malignancy:
   (a) NHL (especially ciclosporin) – many-fold increase
   (b) skin cancer (especially azathioprine) – many-fold increase
   (c) other malignancies – slight increase
2 Cardiovascular: IHD 10–20× more prevalent
3 Infections:
   (a) opportunistic, e.g. PCP, CMV
   (b) may lead to: myocarditis, encephalitis, retinitis, renal function
        deteriorates
4 Recurrence of disease after transplant may occur in:
   (a) focal segmental glomerulosclerosis
   (b) IgA nephropathy

    (c) membranous GN
    (d) mesangiocapillary GN
    (e) Alport's syndrome – anti-GBM disease
    (f) vasculitis (monitor auto-immune antibody levels, e.g. ANCA).

Conditions (a) to (d) are the most likely to recur, but all
glomerulonephritides can recur.

THIRST AND WATER REGULATION

Causes of syndrome of inappropriate ADH production (SIADH)

Malignancy

1 Bronchus, bladder, prostate, pancreas
2 Lymphoma
3 Ewing's sarcoma
4 Mesothelioma
5 Thymoma.

Pulmonary disorders

1 Pneumonia
2 Abscess
3 TB
4 PEEP
5 Asthma.

Central nervous system

1 Encephalitis
2 Meningitis
3 Trauma
4 Acute intermittent porphyria
5 Guillain–Barré syndrome
6 Subarachnoid haemorrhage
7 Hydrocephalus
8 Acute psychosis.

Drugs (see also page 59)

1 Chlorpropamide
2 Carbamazepine
3 Cyclophosphamide
4 Tolbutamide
5 Haloperidol.

Causes of diabetes insipidus (see also page 59)

Cranial causes

1 Idiopathic
2 Craniopharyngioma
3 Infiltrative conditions of the hypothalamus, e.g. sarcoidosis, histiocytosis X
4 Trauma
5 Pituitary surgery
6 Lymphocytic hypophysitis
7 Dysgerminomas.

Nephrogenic causes

Due to decreased action of ADH.

Primary

1 Childhood-onset
2 X-linked/dominant
3 Tubular receptor abnormality.

Secondary

1 Hypercalcaemia
2 Hypokalaemia
3 Renal disease:
   (a) chronic pyelonephritis
   (b) APKD
   (c) post-obstruction
   (d) osmotic
   (e) sarcoid
4 Lithium

5 Demeclocycline
6 Amphotericin.

Investigation of polyuria

1 Record fluid intake
2 Record urine volume
3 Blood glucose, urea and electrolytes, calcium
4 Urinalysis
5 Early-morning urine osmolality
6 Water deprivation test.

Water deprivation test

1 Used to identify the cause of polyuria and/or polydipsia
2 Hourly urine and plasma osmolality measured until 3% of body weight is lost
3 Injection of DDAVP (synthetic ADH) given and hourly urine collections continued.

Table 41

	Initial plasma osmolality	Final urine osmolality (mmol/kg)	Urine osmolality post-DDAVP (mmol/kg)	Final plasma ADH
Normal	Normal	>600	>600	High
Cranial DI	High	<300	>600	Low
Nephrogenic DI	High	<300	<300	High
Primary polydipsia	Low	300–400 (approx.)	400 (approx.)	Moderate
Partial cranial DI	High	300–400	400–600	Relatively low

GLOMERULONEPHRITIS

Screening

1 Stixtesting of urine (protein, haematuria)
2 Quantify proteinuria with 24-hour urine collection
3 Urine microscopy for red cells and casts.

Common renal syndromes

1 Asymptomatic proteinuria: proteinuria <3 g/day
2 Nephrotic syndrome: proteinuria >3 g/day, oedema, serum albumin
   <25 g/l and increased cholesterol
3 Nephritic syndrome: hypertension, haematuria, oedema and oliguria
4 Haematuria: microscopic or macroscopic.

Causes of nephrotic syndrome

1 Primary glomerular disease
2 Diabetes mellitus
3 Infection (malaria, leprosy, hepatitis B)
4 Pre-eclampsia
5 Accelerated hypertension
6 Myeloma
7 Amyloidosis
8 SLE
9 Relapsing polychondritis
10 Drugs:
   (a) gold
   (b) penicillamine
   (c) captopril
   (d) NSAIDs
   (e) mercury
11 Rare causes:
   (a) vesico-ureteric reflux
   (b) constrictive pericarditis
   (c) sickle cell anaemia
   (d) allergies
   (e) 'Finnish type' nephrotic syndrome.

Causes of macroscopic haematuria

1 Urinary tract malignancy
2 Urinary infections
3 Acute GN
4 IgA nephropathy
5 Renal calculi
6 Renal papillary necrosis
7 Prostatic hypertrophy

8 Trauma.

Histological types of glomerulonephritis

Minimal-change GN

1 Presents with nephrotic syndrome
2 More common in children
3 Selective proteinuria
4 Steroid-responsive
5 Electron microscopy shows foot-process fusion
6 Prognosis excellent.

Membranous GN

1 May present as:
    (a) nephrotic syndrome
    (b) proteinuria, or
    (c) chronic renal failure
2 Subepithelial deposits (IgG, complement)
3 'Rule of thirds':
        1/3 progress to CRF and ESRF
        1/3 respond to immunosuppressive therapy
        1/3 remit spontaneously
4 May be idiopathic, or secondary to:
    (a) malignancy (bronchus, stomach, lymphoma, colon, CLL)
    (b) chronic infection (hepatitis B, malaria, syphilis)
    (c) drugs (NSAIDs, gold, penicillamine, captopril)
    (d) connective tissue diseases (SLE, rheumatoid arthritis, MCTD, Sjögren's syndrome)
    (e) sarcoidosis
    (f) Guillaine–Barré syndrome
    (g) primary biliary cirrhosis.

Focal segmental glomerulosclerosis (FSGS)

1 Middle-aged are most commonly affected
2 Presents as proteinuria, nephrotic syndrome
3 Associated with HIV/AIDS
4 IgM deposits in glomerulus
5 25% progress to ESRF.

Mesangioproliferative GN (IgA nephropathy or Berger's disease)

1 Occurs in young adults
2 Presents with haematuria (micro- or macroscopic)
3 Associated with URTI
4 Increased incidence in the Far East
5 50% show increased serum IgA
6 25% progress to ESRF after 20 years
7 Associated with:
   (a) coeliac disease
   (b) dermatitis herpetiformis
   (c) cirrhosis
   (d) mycosis fungoides
   (e) Wiskott–Aldrich syndrome
8 Microscopy shows:
   (a) mesangial cell proliferation
   (b) IgA++ staining.

Mesangiocapillary GN (MCGN)

1 Presents as nephrotic syndrome or proteinuria
2 May be familial – MCGN type 2 is associated with partial lipodystrophy (C3 nephritic factor). Other causes include:
   (a) shunt nephritis
   (b) sickle cell disease
   (c) alpha-1-antitrypsin deficiency
   (d) rheumatoid arthritis
   (e) Kartagener's syndrome
3 Microscopy shows double contour on basement membrane (immune deposition)
4 Poor prognosis – 50% progress to ESRF.

Diffuse proliferative GN

1 May present as nephritic syndrome or ARF
2 Follows streptococcal infection
3 Preceded by sore throat or skin disease (Third-World impetigo)
4 Occurs in children or young adults
5 Low C3.

Rapidly progressive GN (crescentic)

1 Presents with ARF with systemic disease or nephrotic syndrome
2 Vasculitis – ANCA-positive or -negative, SLE, Goodpasture's syndrome (type IV collagen)
3 Microscopy:
   (a) Goodpasture's – linear IgG on basement membrane
   (b) other causes – proliferative lesions and areas of necrosis
   (c) crescent formation
4 Management: immunosuppressant therapy ± plasma exchange
5 Mortality >20%.

GN and hypocomplementaemia

Associated in:
1 SLE
2 Shunt nephritis – coagulase-negative staphylococcal infection of ventriculo-atrial shunts
3 Primary complement deficiency
4 Endocarditis
5 Post-streptococcal GN
6 Mesangiocapillary GN
7 Cryoglobulinaemia type 2.

Goodpasture's syndrome

1 Autoantibody disease
2 Antigen involved is within collagen type IV
3 Ab binds to glomerular and alveolar basement membrane
4 Pathology:
   (a) crescentic GN
   (b) pulmonary haemorrhage
5 Presentation:
   (a) haemoptysis, haematuria
   (b) breathlessness
   (c) massive pulmonary haemorrhage
6 Management:
   (a) steroids
   (b) cyclophosphamide
   (c) plasma exchange
7 Prognosis:

(a) depends on renal function at presentation
(b) poor if ITU care is necessary.

INHERITED RENAL DISEASES

Polycystic kidney disease

1 Autosomal dominant
2 *PKD1* on chromosome 16 (86%); *PKD2* on chromosome 4 (10%)
3 Cysts develop in teenage years
4 Presentation varies
5 Associations:
   (a) liver cysts
   (b) berry aneurysms
   (c) malignant change
   (d) pancreatic cysts
   (e) MV prolapse or AR
   (f) hepatic fibrosis
   (g) diverticular disease.

Alport's syndrome

1 85% are X-linked dominant
2 Microscopy shows variable thickness and splitting of glomerular basement membrane
3 Presents with:
   (a) deafness
   (b) microscopic haematuria
   (c) proteinuria
   (d) CRF
   (e) nephrotic syndrome in one-third
4 Males all develop renal failure; females show minor abnormalities only
5 Gene involved codes alpha-5 chain of type IV collagen.

INTERSTITIAL NEPHRITIS

Acute interstitial nephritis

Presentation

1 Mild renal impairment
2 Hypertension
3 Interstitial oedema on biopsy with acute tubular necrosis.

Causes

1 Idiopathic
2 Infection:
  (a) leptospirosis
  (b) mycobacterial
3 Drugs:
  (a) rifampicin
  (b) NSAIDs
  (c) furosemide (frusemide)
  (d) cephalosporins
  (e) penicillins
  (f) sulphonamides
  (g) allopurinol
  (h) thiazides
  (i) cimetidine.

Treatment

1 Remove the cause, e.g. drugs
2 Some require a small dose of steroids.

Most make a complete recovery.

Chronic interstitial nephritis

Presentation

1 CRF
2 ESRF
3 RTA type 1
4 Nephrogenic diabetes insipidus

5 Salt-wasting states
6 Biopsy shows chronic inflammation, scarring, tubule loss.

Causes

1 SLE
2 Rheumatoid arthritis
3 Myeloma
4 Light-chain nephropathy
5 Sickle cell disease
6 Lead
7 Cadmium
8 Hypercalcaemia
9 Hypokalaemia
10 Hyperuricaemia
11 Irradiation
12 Chronic transplant rejection
13 Wegener's granulomatosis
14 Tuberculosis
15 Sarcoidosis
16 Chronic pyelonephritis
17 Alport's syndrome
18 Balkan nephropathy
19 Drugs:
    (a) ciclosporin A
    (b) cisplatin
    (c) lithium
    (d) iron
    (e) analgesics.

Analgesic nephropathy

1 Due to chronic analgesic usage
2 'Cup and spill' calyces on IVU
3 Papillary necrosis
4 Incidence is decreasing.

Treatment

As in the acute form. Steroids may be beneficial.

RENAL CALCULI

Prevalence is 3% in the UK. Calcium-containing calculi are the most common.

Predisposing factors

Metabolic

1 Hypercalciuria
2 Primary hypercalcaemia
3 Renal tubular acidosis
4 Uric aciduria
5 Hyperoxaluria
6 Increased oxalate intake
7 Cystinuria.

Structural

1 Polcystic kidney disease
2 Reflux nephropathy
3 Nephrocalcinosis
4 Medullary sponge kidney.

Other factors

1 Dehydration
2 Cadmium
3 Beryllium
4 Triamterene.

Treatment

1 Increase fluid intake
2 Decrease protein in the diet
3 Treat underlying causes
4 Thiazide diuretics
5 Stone removal and/or lithotripsy.

SYSTEMIC DISORDERS AND THE KIDNEY

Amyloidosis

Chronic infiltrative disorders characterised by deposition of extracellular fibrillar material (i.e. amyloid).

Types of amyloidosis

Classification is based on the type of amyloid protein found:
1 Primary amyloid (AL)
2 Secondary amyloid (AA or AL)
3 Senile amyloid (pre-albumin)
4 Dialysis amyloid (β_2-microglobulin).

Presentation

1 Proteinuria (asymptomatic to nephrotic)
2 Chronic renal failure.

Investigation

1 Histology: Congo-red stain on biopsy
2 SAP (Serum Amybid P) scan.

Treatment

1 Remove or treat any underlying cause
2 Cytotoxic therapy
3 Bone marrow transplant.

Prognosis

1 Six-year survival on dialysis is 44%
   (a) patients on dialysis
   (b) faster speed of onset
   (c) multisystem involvement.

Clinical features of systemic amyloidosis

1 Hepatosplenomegaly
2 Nephrotic syndrome

3 Renal failure
4 Macroglossia
5 GI bleeding
6 Malabsorption
7 Restrictive cardiomyopathy
8 Congestive cardiomyopathy
9 Skin deposition
10 Neuropathy
11 Bleeding disorder.

Associations of secondary amyloidosis

1 Familial Mediterranean fever
2 Rheumatoid arthritis
3 Psoriatic arthritis
4 Ankylosing spondylitis
5 Sjögrens's syndrome
6 Behçet's syndrome
7 Reiter's syndrome
8 Juvenile rheumatoid
9 Whipple's disease
10 Inflammatory bowel disease
11 Polymyositis
12 Scleroderma
13 Tuberculosis
14 Osteomyelitis
15 Paraplegia
16 Heroin abuse
17 Leprosy
18 Syphilis
19 Bronchiectasis
20 Myeloma
21 Renal cell carcinoma.

Renovascular disease

Associated with general vascular disease. Co-morbidity is high and so prognosis is poor.

Presentation

1 Hypertension
2 Flash pulmonary oedema
3 End-stage renal failure (ESRF)
4 CRF
5 ARF following ACE inhibitor or angiotensin-II antagonist.

Investigation

1 Asymmetrical kidneys on ultrasound scan
2 Captopril renogram
3 Magnetic resonance angiogram
4 Conventional angiography.

Treatment

1 Angioplasty ± stenting
2 Aspirin
3 Lipid-lowering treatment.

Connective tissue disorders

Renal disease is associated with:
1 Rheumatoid arthritis
2 Mixed connective tissue disease
3 Sjögren's syndrome
4 Systemic sclerosis
5 Systemic lupus erythematosus.

SLE nephritis

1 40% have renal involvement
2 Women : men ratio is 10 : 1
3 Any presentation possible
4 Histology variable, but 'wire-loop' lesions are characteristic
5 Treatment:
   (a) ARF and SLE – aggressive immunosuppressant therapy with pulsed methylprednisolone and intravenous cyclophosphamide then high-dose oral prednisolone
   (b) maintenance with oral steroids and azathioprine

(c) plasma exchange if severe or with pulmonary haemorrhage.

Systemic sclerosis

1 Presentation:
   (a) accelerated hypertension
   (b) micro-angiopathic haemolytic anaemia (MAHA)
   (c) acute renal failure
2 Histology: onion-skin appearance of interlobular arteries
3 Treatment: ACE inhibitor for hypertension
4 Prognosis: poor due to involvement of other organs. Many progress to ESRF.

Diabetes mellitus (DM)

Most common cause of ESRF in the UK. Renal disease present in 49% of type 1 diabetics 20–40 years from diagnosis of DM.

Presentation

1 Microalbuminuria (30–250 mg/day)
2 Proteinuria (>0.5 g/day)
3 Hypertension
4 Nephrotic syndrome
5 Chronic renal failure.

Biopsy findings

1 Kimmelstiel–Wilson nodules are characteristic
2 Mesangial expansion
3 Diffuse glomerular sclerosis.

Treatment

1 ACE inhibitors and angiotensin blockers
2 Tight glycaemic control
3 Tight control of blood pressure (target is $<130/75$).

Prognosis

Established nephropathy proceeds to ESRF. Prognosis is poor due to co-morbidity, e.g. cardiovascular disease.

Hypertension (see also page 33)

Primary hypertension

1 Renal damage common
2 May present with proteinuria and/or chronic renal failure, or with acute renal failure
3 Biopsy findings:
   (a) arterial fibrinoid necrosis
   (b) severe tubular and glomerular ischaemia (ARF)
   (c) interstitial fibrosis and glomerulosclerosis (CRF).

Secondary hypertension

1 Hypertension is due to renal disease in 4% of all hypertensive patients
2 Other causes (1% of all hypertensive patients):
   (a) coarctation of the aorta
   (b) endocrine:
      (i) Cushing's syndrome
      (ii) acromegaly
      (iii) Conn's syndrome
      (iv) phaeochromocytoma
   (c) alcohol
   (d) obesity.

Myeloma

May cause:
1 Acute renal failure: light chain nephropathy, increased uric acid, increased calcium may contribute. May be reversible with chemotherapy, rehydration
2 Chronic renal failure:
   (a) amyloidosis
   (b) chronic interstitial nephritis
   (c) cast nephropathy
   (d) usually progresses to ESRF
3 Light chain nephropathy:
   (a) kappa and lambda chains
   (b) direct toxicity
   (c) cast formation
   (d) acute tubular necrosis

(e) tubular atrophy.

Vasculitis (see also pages 414–418)

Inflammation of blood vessels, classified in terms of size of vessel involved.

Wegener's granulomatosis

1 Small vessels with granulomas
2 Focal necrotising and crescentic GN
3 cANCA positive
4 Other systems involved:
   (a) cavitating pulmonary nodules and haemoptysis
   (b) upper respiratory tract
   (c) eye
   (d) cutaneous vasculitis
   (e) GI tract
   (f) peripheral nerves.

Microscopic polyangiitis

1 Small-vessel vasculitis
2 Focal necrotising and crescentic GN
3 Resembles Wegener's
4 cANCA or pANCA positive
5 Other systems involved:
   (a) pulmonary involvement with haemorrhage
   (b) episcleritis
   (c) skin
   (d) GI tract
   (e) peripheral nerves.

Polyarteritis nodosa (PAN)

1 Medium vessels involved
2 Microaneurysms
3 Renal infarcts
4 Usually ANCA negative
5 Other systems involved:

(a) pulmonary
(b) GI tract
(c) peripheral nerves.

Churg–Strauss disease

1 Medium vessels involved with granulomas
2 ANCA positive or negative
3 Renal vasculitis
4 Other systems involved:
    (a) pulmonary infiltrates and asthma
    (b) eosinophilia
    (c) peripheral nerves.

Henoch–Schönlein purpura

1 Small vessels involved (IgA deposition)
2 Mesangial hypercellularity to crescentic GN
3 ANCA negative
4 Cutaneous involvement.

Treatment of vasculitis

Aggressive immunosuppression required:
1 Initial treatment:
    (a) pulsed methylprednisolone and cyclophosphamide
    (b) high-dose steroids
2 Maintenance:
    (a) steroids
    (b) azathioprine
3 Plasma exchange may be necessary.

NEPHROTOXIC DRUGS (see also pages 49–50)

Drugs that cause tubule damage

Usually results in acute tubular necrosis.
1 Aminoglycosides
2 Cisplatin
3 Amphotericin.

Drugs that affect blood supply

1 Ciclosporin: causes arterial damage
2 ACE inhibitors: RAA system dependent
3 NSAIDs: alter prostaglandin metabolism.

Drugs that cause glomerulonephritis

1 Gold: immune complex GN, usually membranous
2 Penicillamine: membranous GN, delayed response.

RADIOCONTRAST NEPHROPATHY

Risk factors:
1 Hypovolaemia
2 Diabetes mellitus
3 Pre-existing CRF
4 Hypercalcaemia
5 Hyperuricaemia
6 Older age
7 Myeloma
8 High contrast dose
9 Contrast with high iodine content.

TUMOURS OF THE RENAL TRACT

Benign

1 Adenoma
2 Hamartoma
3 Renin-secreting (juxtaglomerular cell).

Renal cell carcinoma

1 Arises from tubular epithelium
2 Renal vein invasion
3 Pulmonary emboli
4 A cause of pyrexia of unknown origin
5 Left testicular vein occlusion leads to a left-sided varicocele

6 Polycythaemia (erythropoietin production)
7 Hypercalcaemia (PTH-like molecule)
8 Hypertension (renin secretion)
9 Cushing's syndrome (ACTH production)
10 Prognosis: 50% five-year survival rate.

Wilms' tumour

1 Childhood tumour
2 Arises from embryonic renal tissue
3 Early metastasis
4 Treatment: nephrectomy and actinomycin D
5 Prognosis: 65% three-year survival rate.

Urothelial tumours

1 Transitional cell origin
2 Commonly present with bleeding
3 Urinary tract obstruction may occur
4 Often multiple
5 Associations:
  (a) smoking
  (b) analgesic nephropathy
  (c) exposure to rubber or aniline dye
  (d) renal calculi
  (e) cystic kidney disease
  (f) chronic cystitis
  (g) *Schistosoma* infection
6 Treatment:
  (a) nephroureterectomy (lesion in renal pelvis or ureter) or
  (b) cystectomy (bladder), plus
  (c) radiotherapy
7 Prognosis: 50% five-year survival rate.

Neurology

INTERPRETING CEREBRAL LESIONS

The cerebral cortex

1 Motor – precentral gyrus (frontal lobe)
2 Somatosensory – postcentral gyrus:
    (a) auditory – superior temporal lobe
    (b) visual – occipital cortex (calcarine sulcus)
    (c) olfactory – frontal lobe (orbitofrontal cortex)
    (d) Broca's area – dominant frontal lobe, speech output
    (e) Wernicke's area – dominant posterior superior temporal gyrus, word comprehension.

Frontal lobe

Lesions in frontal lobe may result in:
1 Personality change – apathetic or disinhibited
2 Broca's aphasia – ('telegraphic' output)
3 Anosmia
4 Abnormal affective reactions
5 Difficulty with planning or maintaining motivation
6 Primitive reflexes (e.g. grasp, rooting, pout)
7 Perseveration.

Parietal lobe

Parietal lobe damage may result in:
    1 All the 'A's . . .
    2 Apraxia
    3 Acalculia
    4 Agraphia
    5 Drawing apraxia

6 Constructional apraxia (nondominant)
7 Visual field defects – usually homogeneous inferior quadrantanopia
8 Anosognosia (denial of illness, non-down)
9 Visuospatial neglect or extinction
10 Astereognosis (failure to recognise common objects by touch)
11 Gerstmann's syndrome:
  (a) alexia (inability to read)
  (b) agraphia (inability to write)
  (c) R/L confusion
  (d) finger agnosia.

Occipital lobe

Occipital lesions may result in:
1 Cortical blindness
2 Homonymous hemianopia
3 Visual agnosia (inability to comprehend meaning of objects)
4 Specific visual processing defects:
  (a) akinetopsia – impaired perception of motion
  (b) achromatopsia – impaired perception of colours.

Temporal lobe

The following conditions may result from temporal lobe lesions:
1 Wernicke's aphasia
2 Cortical deafness (auditory cortex – bilateral)
3 Auditory agnosia
4 Memory impairment
5 Impaired musical perception
6 Emotional disturbance (limbic cortex damage)
7 Visual field defect – homonymous superior quadrantanopia (lower loop optic radiation).

DEMENTIA (see also pages 358–360)

1 An acquired, global impairment of intellect, memory and personality
2 Usually untreatable and progressive
3 Other conditions may mimic dementia:
  (a) depression

(b) postictal
(c) acute confusion
(d) psychosis of old age.

Causes of dementia

1 Alzheimer's disease
2 Multi-infarct disease
3 Pick's disease
4 Huntington's disease
5 Parkinson's disease
6 Creutzfeld–Jakob disease (CJD)
7 Lewy-body dementia
8 AIDS-associated
9 Chronic drug intoxication
10 Acute or chronic head injury
11 Chronic alcoholism
12 Tumours, primary or secondary.

Potentially treatable causes of dementia

1 B_{12} deficiency
2 Folate deficiency
3 Wilson's disease
4 Hypothyroidism
5 Niacin deficiency
6 Normal-pressure hydrocephalus.

Alzheimer's disease

1 Short-term memory problems
2 Disorientation
3 Personality changes
4 Cognitive impairment
5 Progressive decline.

Pathology

1 Senile plaques (β-amyloid)
2 Neurofibrillary tangles (tau protein)
3 Hippocampus particularly affected

4 Loss of:
   (a) cholinergic neurones
   (b) choline acetyl transferase activity.

Chromosomal associations

1 5% are familial
2 Link with Down's syndrome (chromosome 21)
3 Apolipoprotein E (chromsome 19).

Pick's disease

1 Focal lobar atrophy
2 Frontotemporal functional deterioration
3 Pick bodies in cellular cytoplasm
4 Progressive language disturbance (expressive)
5 Prominent frontal lobe features.

Creutzfeldt–Jakob disease (CJD)

A prion disease. Prion proteins are normal membrane-bound, cellular products. CJD is caused by the accumulation of an abnormal isoform of the glycoprotein.
Other prion diseases:
1 Kuru (Papua New Guinea) transmitted by eating human brain tissue
2 Gerstmann–Straussler–Scheinker disease
3 Fatal familial insomnia.

CJD has inherited, acquired and sporadic forms:
1 Inherited:
   (a) autosomnal dominant
   (b) PRNP gene
   (c) chromosome 20
2 Acquired, due to:
   (a) altered prion protein introduced into host
   (b) modification of host-native prion protein into the abnormal form
   (c) infectious agent resistant to heat, irradiation, autoclaving
3 Sporadic:
   (a) 85% of all cases
   (b) incidence one in a million worldwide

(c) mean age 65 years
(d) bovine spongiform encephalopathy-agent related (BSE).

Clinical features

1 Rapidly progressive dementia
2 Myoclonus
3 Biphasic high-amplitude sharp waves on EEG.

New variant (nv)CJD

1 Younger age of onset (median age at death 29 years)
2 EEG features absent
3 Atypical clinical presentation
4 Behavioural disturbance
5 Psychiatric disturbance.

CEREBROVASCULAR DISEASE

Transient ischaemic attacks (TIAs)

1 Focal CNS disturbance
2 Develops in minutes/hours
3 Full recovery within 24 hours of onset.

Differential diagnosis

1 Epilepsy
2 Migraine
3 Hypoglycaemia
4 Malignant hypertension
5 Multiple sclerosis
6 Transient global amnesia
7 Ménière's disease and benign positional vertigo
8 Peripheral nerve entrapment.

Stroke (cerebrovascular accident, CVA)

1 Clinically, as for TIA but deficit persists
2 Causes:

(a) embolic
(b) thrombotic
(c) haemorrhagic
3 Clinical presentation depends on vascular territory affected.

Lacunar infarctions

1 Pure motor, sensorimotor or sensory involvement
2 No higher cortical functions affected
3 Hypertension-associated
4 Anterior cerebral circulation
5 Posterior cerebral circulation
6 Associated with a better prognosis.

Modifiable risk factors for TIA and stroke (see also page 30)

1 Diabetes
2 Hypertension
3 Smoking
4 Previous TIA or CVA
5 Male sex
6 Family history
7 Drug use (e.g. alcohol, oral contraceptive pill (OCP), illicit drugs)
8 Raised haemoglobin.

Investigation and management of TIA and stroke

Diagnosis

1 Clinical
2 CT scan of brain
3 MRI scan considered if there are cerebellar symptoms and CT is normal
4 Investigation of risk factors:
    (a) hypercholesterolaemia
    (b) carotid stenosis – carotid Doppler
    (c) hypertension
    (d) diabetes
    (e) cardiac source – echocardiogram.

Treatment/secondary prevention

1 Conservative

2 Aspirin or anticoagulation (if not haemorrhagic) for secondary
  prevention
3 Mortality 20–30%
4 Carotid endarterectomy.

Prognosis

1 25–30% remain significantly disabled
2 Lacunar infarcts have a better prognosis
3 Poor outcome associated with:
   (a) greater age
   (b) coma at onset
   (c) persistent neglect.

Subarachnoid haemorrhage (SAH)

Accounts for 5–10% of all strokes.

Causes

1 Rupture of aneurysm – 80% are of anterior circulation (mainly anterior
  communicating artery)
2 Arterio-venous malformation
3 Trauma
4 Cocaine or amphetamine abuse
5 Hypertension
6 Spontaneous.

Present with headache and/or coma.

Investigation and management

1 *Diagnosis:*
   (a) CT scan
   (b) lumbar puncture:
       (i) xanthochromia (more than 4 hours post-episode)
       (ii) raised blood cell count on microscopy
2 *Treatment:*
   (a) nimodipine – reduces vasospasm
   (b) neurosurgical clipping of aneurysm
3 *Prognosis:* 30% mortality from first episode

4 *Complications:*
  (a) vasospasm – ischaemic injury
  (b) 30% re-bleed
  (c) hydrocephalus
  (d) SIADH
  (e) fever
  (f) 30% recover to be independent.

Associations with intracerebral aneurysms

1 Polycystic kidney disease
2 Ehlers–Danlos syndrome
3 Medium-vessel vasculitis (e.g. polyarteritis nodosa)
4 Coarctation of the aorta
5 Fibromuscular dysplasia causing renal artery stenosis.

Lateral medullary syndrome (Wallenberg's syndrome)

1 Vertebral artery or posterior inferior cerebellar artery occlusion
2 Ipsilateral pain and temperature loss on the face (fifth cranial nerve)
3 Ipsilateral paralysis of palate, pharynx, vocal cords (ninth and tenth cranial nerves)
4 Ipsilateral ataxia
5 Contralateral pain and temperature loss on the body (spinothalamic tract)
6 Ipsilateral Horner's syndrome (descending sympathetic outflow)
7 Vertigo, nausea and vomiting, nystagmus (vestibular nuclei).

VIRAL ENCEPHALITIS (see also page 246)

1 Confusion
2 Altered conscious level
3 Seizures
4 Focal neurology.

Causes

1 Herpes simplex virus
2 Mumps virus
3 Varicella zoster virus

4 EBV
5 Coxsackievirus
6 Echoviruses.

Herpes simplex encephalitis

1 Anterior temporal lobe pathology
2 CSF lymphocytosis
3 Low CSF glucose (20%)
4 CSF protein concentration raised
5 EEG – focal temporal lobe involvement
6 Treat with aciclovir.

EPILEPSY

1 Paroxysmal discharge of neurones
2 More than one seizure
3 Prevalence 0.7%, constant at all ages
4 Incidence greatest in young and elderly.

Types of epilepsy

1 *Simple partial seizures:*
   (a) consciousness intact
   (b) EEG – local discharge in corresponding area
   (c) may progress
2 *Complex partial seizures:*
   (a) consciousness impaired
   (b) medial temporal focus
   (c) aura – déjà vu, strong smell, or rising sensation in abdomen
   (d) automatisms
3 *Tonic clonic seizures:*
   (a) loss of consciousness
   (b) short tonic phase then clonic movements
   (c) no warning
   (d) incontinence
   (e) postictal confusion.

Treatment of epilepsy

Recent developments in the therapeutics of epilepsy have concentrated on agents which interact with neurotransmitters.

1 Glutamic acid is an excitatory central nervous system neurotransmitter; **lamotrigine** inhibits it, so suppressing seizures. The side-effects of lamotrigine include mood changes, maculopapular rashes, influenza-like symptoms and Stevens–Johnson syndrome
2 Gamma amino butyric acid (GABA) is an inhibitory central nervous system neurotransmitter. Gabapentin and vigabatrin potentiate GABA and thus may be used to treat seizures
3 **Vigabatrin** is used for refractory epilepsy, potentiating GABA by irreversible inhibition of GABA transaminase. Side-effects of vigabatrin include mood disturbance and psychosis in 5%. Severe visual field defects may occur from one month to several years afer initiation of therapy; regular visual field assessment is advised
4 **Diazepam** also terminates seizures by indrectly interacting with GABA transmission. It stimulates the benzodiazepine receptor in the brain which in turn enhances the affinity of the neighbouring GABA receptor for its neurotransmitter
5 **Carbamazepine** is a derivative of the tricylic antidepressants and is useful for epilepsy and also neural pain (e.g. trigeminal or post-herpetic neuralgia). Patients commonly experience headaches and diplopia on starting carbamazepine and 5–15% of patients can develop a generalized morbilliform rash
6 **Sodium valproate** is used in absence attacks and temporal lobe epilepsy. It inhibits liver enzymes and may potentiate other anti-epileptics such a phenytoin. It may cause alopecia, with curly regrowth after stopping the drug.

Driving and epilepsy

1 After one seizure patients are not permitted to drive for one year
2 Established epilepsy – able to drive if:
   (a) fit-free while awake, for 12 months
   (b) attacks only occur while asleep and there have been no attacks for three years
3 HGV licence – for 10 years, must:
   (a) be free of attacks
   (b) be off all medication

(c) have no structural cause.

Pregnancy and epilepsy

1 Seizure rate predicted by rate prior to pregnancy
2 Drugs all have teratogenic effects
3 Epileptic drugs not contraindicated
4 Risks of uncontrolled epilepsy greater than effects of drugs
5 Current drug used if starting treatment is lamotrigine
6 Folic acid supplements decrease malformation.

HYDROCEPHALUS

Normal-pressure hydrocephalus

1 Presents with classic triad of symptoms:
   (a) dementia
   (b) gait abnormality
   (c) urinary incontinence (frontal lobe)
2 May mimic Parkinson's disease
3 Defect of CSF absorption, basal meningeal thickening
4 May be secondary to:
   (a) meningitis
   (b) head injury
   (c) subarachnoid haemorrhage.
5 Radiology:
   (a) dilated ventricles
   (b) hydrocephalus
   (c) pressure only high intermittently
6 No papilloedema seen
7 Treatment – ventriculo-peritoneal shunt may help.

Benign intracranial hypertension

1 Headache
2 Papilloedema
3 No focal neurology
4 Brain scan normal
5 CSF pressure increased
6 Overweight young women

7 *Treatment:*
   (a) weight loss
   (b) sequential lumbar puncture
   (c) acetazolamide
   (d) ventriculo-peritoneal shunt.

Causes

Iatrogenic:
1 OCP
2 Nalidixic acid
3 Nitrofurantoins
4 Steroids
5 Vitamin A
6 Tetracycline.

WERNICKE'S ENCEPHALOPATHY (see also page 356)

1 Acute onset
2 *Clinical features:*
   (a) ataxia
   (b) nystagamus
   (c) ophthalmoplegia
   (d) global confusional state
   (e) neuropathy
3 *Causes:*
   (a) alcohol
   (b) hyperemesis gravidarum
   (c) dialysis
   (d) gastrointestinal causes
4 Treat with thiamine
5 May lead to Korsakoff's syndrome.

THE SPINAL CORD AND PERIPHERAL NERVES

Carpal tunnel syndrome

1 Median nerve

2 Numbness and dysaesthesia (radial three-and-a-half fingers)
3 Weakness of muscles (**LOAF**):
  (a) **l**ateral two lumbricals
  (b) **o**pponens pollicis
  (c) **a**bductor pollicis
  (d) **f**lexor pollicis brevis
4 *Associations:*
  (a) pregnancy
  (b) obesity
  (c) hypothyroidism
  (d) acromegaly
  (e) amyloidosis
  (f) rheumatoid arthritis
5 *Treatment:*
  (a) splinting of the wrist
  (b) diuretics
  (c) steroid injection to flexor retinaculum
  (d) surgical decompression.

Ulnar nerve

Serves the muscles of the hypothenar eminence.
1 Abductor digiti minimi
2 Median two lumbricals
3 All interossei.

Radial nerve

1 No muscles of the hand
2 Exterior compartment of the forearm.

Causes of wasting of the small muscles of the hand

1 Arthritis
2 Motor neurone disease
3 Syringomyelia
4 Polyneuropathy
5 Brachial plexus injury
6 Other cervical cord pathology.

Common peroneal nerve palsy

Presents with:
1 Foot drop
2 Weakness of inversion of the foot (L4)
3 Weakness of dorsiflexion, tibialis anterior (L5)
4 Weakness of eversion, peronei (S1)
5 Sensory loss dorsum of the foot.

L5 root lesion – eversion remains intact.

Causes

1 Compression at the head of the fibula
2 Weight loss
3 Diabetes mellitus
4 Polyartertis nodosa
5 Leprosy
6 Collagen-vascular diseases.

Polyneuropathies

Mainly sensory

1 Leprosy
2 Diabetes mellitus
3 Amyloidosis
4 Vitamin B_{12} deficiency
5 Hereditary sensory neuropathy
6 Carcinoma
7 Uraemia.

Mainly motor

1 Guillain–Barré syndrome
2 Porphyria
3 Lead intoxication
4 Diphtheria
5 Hereditary sensory and motor neuropathy (HSMN) types I and II
6 Chronic inflammatory demyelinating polyneuropathy (CIDP).

Autonomic neuropathy

Presents with:
1 Postural hypotension
2 Sluggish or absent pupillary light response
3 Anhidrosis
4 Defective piloerection
5 Impotence
6 Urinary incontinence
7 Nocturnal diarrhoea
8 Constipation
9 Absent cardiovascular responses.

Causes

1 Diabetes mellitus
2 Gullain–Barré syndrome
3 Amyloidosis
4 Chronic liver failure
5 Renal failure
6 Multiple nervous system atrophies (e.g. Shy–Drager syndrome).

Guillain–Barré syndrome (GBS)

1 Acute infective polyneuropathy
2 Muscle weakness:
    (a) ascending
    (b) symmetrical
    (c) progressive
    (d) leads to paralysis
3 Association with previous infection – respiratory or gastointestinal, e.g. CMV
4 Immunological response to preceding infection
5 Diagnostic features:
    (a) areflexia in more than one limb
    (b) progression in less than four weeks
    (c) no evidence of toxic exposure or botulism.
6 Investigation findings:
    (a) raised CSF proteins
    (b) normal CSF white cell count
    (c) slowing of nerve conduction

NEUROLOGY

     (d) EMG shows denervation
7 *Prognosis* poor with:
     (a) older age
     (b) rapid onset of symptoms
     (c) axonal neuropathy on nerve conduction studies
     (d) *Campylobacter jejuni* infection
8 *Treatment:*
     (a) intravenous immunoglobulins
     (b) plasma exchange
     (c) respiratory care:
        (i) monitor vital capacity four-hourly
        (ii) counting 1–20 in one breath?
        (iii) may reuire artificial ventilation.

Miller Fisher syndrome

1 Variant of GBS
2 Ophthalmoplegia
3 Ataxia
4 Areflexia.

Motor neurone disease (MND)

1 Progressive neurodegenerative disease
2 Usually sporadic
3 Familial in 5–10% – SOD I gene on chromosome 21
4 Three patterns of disease:
     (a) *progressive muscular atrophy:*
        (i) 10% show only lower motor neurone signs
        (ii) better prognosis than classical MND
     (b) *progressive bulbar palsy:*
        (i) bulbar musculature
        (ii) 20% present in this manner
        (iii) poor prognosis
     (c) *primary lateral sclerosis:*
        (i) slowly progressive spasticity and weakness of limbs
        (ii) more marked in the legs
        (iii) associated with pseudobulbar palsy
        (iv) variant of MND but better prognosis
5 *Presentation:*

(a) limb weakness:
 (i) foot drop
 (ii) fine movement of hands impaired
 (iii) localised wasting
 (iv) fasciculation
(b) Bulbar symptoms:
 (i) nasal speech (bulbar palsy)
 (ii) spastic dysarthria (pseudobulbar palsy)
 (iii) dysphagia
(c) respiratory failure
(d) parasthesiae (sensory examination normal)
(e) dementia (frontal-lobe type)
6 *Investigations:*
 (a) diagnosis is clinical
 (b) electromyography and nerve conduction studies reveal anterior horn damage
 (c) MRI of spinal cord to rule out other causes, e.g. compressive lesion in the neck
7 *Prognosis* – average life expectancy is:
 (a) two years with bulbar symptoms
 (b) four years with peripheral symptoms.

Causes of fasciculation

1 Motor neurone disease
2 Syringomyelia
3 Thyrotoxicosis
4 Cervical spondylosis
5 Acute poliomyelitis
6 Hyponatraemia
7 Hypomagnesaemia
8 Drugs:
 (a) clofilorate
 (b) lithium
 (c) salbutamol
 (d) anticholinesterase.

Functional anatomy of the spinal cord

1 Corticospinal tract:
   (a) descending
   (b) crosses in midbrain
2 Two ascending pathways:
   (a) dorsal columns:
      (i) joint position sense and vibration sense
      (ii) synapse in brainstem then decussate
   (b) spinothalamic tracts:
      (i) pain and temperature sense
      (ii) cross immediately or within few segments
      (iii) lamination of fibres.

Anterior cord syndrome

1 Artery of Adamkiewicz
2 Flaccid/spastic paraparesis
3 Loss of pain and temperature sensation bilaterally
4 Dorsal columns intact.

Brown–Séquard syndrome

1 Lateral hemisection of cord
2 Ipsilateral upper motor neurone weakness below the lesion
3 Contralateral pain and temperature loss
4 Ipsilateral joint position sense and vibration loss.

Tabes dorsalis

Dorsal root lesion:
1 Joint position sense and pain fibres affected
2 Secondary degeneration of dorsal columns
3 Loss of reflex arc.

Subacute combined degeneration of the cord

Dorsal colum disease.
1 Sensory ataxia
2 Peripheral neuropathy
3 Corticospinal tract – spastic paraparesis

4 Absent knee jerk
5 Extensor plantars.

Absent knee jerks and exterior plantars

1 Friedreich's ataxia
2 Motor neurone disease
3 Taboparesis (neurosyphilis)
4 Vitamin B_{12} deficiency
5 Conus medullaris lesion
6 Diabetes mellitus.

THE CRANIAL NERVES

Optic nerve and visual fields

The visual fields and retina have an inverted and reversed relationship.

Visual field loss

1 Central scotoma ipsilateral optic nerve disease, e.g. neuritis
2 Ipsilateral loss (complete) – optic nerve transection
3 Bitemporal hemianopia – chiasmal lesion:
  (a) craniopharyngioma
  (b) pituitary tumour
  (c) intracranial aneurysm
  (d) meningioma
  (e) dilated third ventricle
4 Homonymous superior quadrantanopia – temporal lobe lesion
5 Homonymous inferior quadrantanopia – parietal lobe lesion
6 Homonymous hemianopia – less congruous – more anterior lesion
7 Homonymous hemianopia – highly congruous – posterior lesion.

The pupil

1 Pupilloconstrictor (parasympathetic) fibres
2 Pupillodilator (sympathetic) fibres
3 Pupillary light reflex:
  (a) afferent: retina, optic nerve, lateral geniculate body, midbrain
  (b) efferent: Edinger–Westphal nucleus (midbrain), third nerve.

Causes of small pupil (miosis)

1 Horner's syndrome
2 Argyll Robertson pupil (do not react to light but normal accommodation reaction)
3 Pontine haemorrhage
4 Myotonic dystrophy
5 Senile miosis
6 Drugs, e.g. opiates, pilocarpine.

Horner's syndrome

1 Miosis
2 Enophthalmos
3 Ptosis (muscle of Muller)
4 Anhidrosis
5 More common in women.

Causes

1 Lesion of the brainstem or spinal cord:
   (a) vascular
   (b) trauma
   (c) neoplastic
   (d) demyelination
   (e) syringomyelia.
2 Preganglonic lesion:
   (a) chest – carcinoma, cervical rib, mediastinal mass
   (b) cervical – lymphadenopathy, trauma, thyroid neoplasm
   (c) surgical – thyroidectomy, carotid angiography, endarterectomy
3 Postganglonic lesion:
   (a) internal carotid artery dissection
   (b) cavernous sinus lesion
   (c) orbital apex disease.

Causes of large pupil (mydriasis)

1 Adie's pupil – idiopathic, reacts poorly to light. Decreased tendon reflexes (Holmes–Adie pupil)
2 Third nerve palsy
3 Drugs – amphetamines, antidepressants, tropicamide, atropine
4 Trauma.

Oculomotor nerves

Innervation

Sixth cranial nerve – lateral rectus
Fourth cranial nerve – superior oblique
Third cranial nerve – the rest
Mnenomic: $LR_6(SO_4)_3$.

Third nerve palsy

1 Ptosis
2 Inability to move the eye superiorly, inferiorly or medially
3 Eye: down and out
4 Pupil fixed and dilated.

Causes

1 Diabetes mellitus
2 Arteriosclerotic
3 Posterior communicating artery aneurysm
4 Cavernous sinus thrombosis, aneurysm or fistula
5 Orbital tumour
6 Thyroid eye disease
7 Trauma
8 Uncal herniation.

Causes of ptosis

(Please see Ophthalmology chapter.)

Fourth nerve palsy

1 Exits dorsal aspect of the brainstem (the only one to do so)
2 Vertical diplopia
3 Noticed when descending stairs or reading.

Causes

1 Diabetes mellitus
2 Vascular
3 Vasculitis

4 Trauma
5 Congenital
6 Cavernous sinus syndrome
7 Orbital apex syndrome.

Sixth nerve palsy

1 Diplopia on lateral gaze
2 Affected eye deviates medially.

Causes

1 Vascular
2 Trauma
3 Cavernous sinus
4 Orbital apex disease
5 Raised intracranial pressure (a false localising sign).

Internuclear ophthalmoplegia

1 Interference in conjugate eye movement
2 Lesion in medial longitudinal fasciculus which connects third and fourth nuclei in the pons.
3 Adduction of eye ipsilateral to lesion impaired
4 Horizontal nystagmus in abducting eye contralateral to lesion
5 Normal convergence
6 May have nystagmus on vertical gaze.

Causes

1 Multiple sclerosis
2 Vascular
3 Trauma
4 Basilar artery occlusion
5 SLE
6 Miller Fisher syndrome
7 Drug overdose (barbiturates, phenytoin or amitryptyline)
8 Wernicke's encephalopathy.

Impaired vertical conjugate gaze

1 Progressive supranuclear palsy

2 Thyroid opththalmopathy
3 Myasthenia gravis
4 Miller Fisher syndrome
5 Parinaud's syndrome – damage to midbrain and superior colliculi.

Nystagmus

A problem with the control of ocular position. There are three types:
1 Pendular – no fast or slow phase
2 Jerk:
    (a) distinct fast/slow components
    (b) amplitude increases on gaze towards the fast phase direction
3 Rotatory – combined horizontal and vertical nystagmus.

Congenital nystagmus

1 X-linked or autosomnal dominant
2 Secondary to poor vision, e.g. cataract, albinism.

Acquired nystagmus

1 Vestibular – fast phase away from the side of the lesion
2 Cerebellar – fast phase towards the side of the lesion
3 Drug-induced – alcohol, barbiturates, phenytoin.

Causes of cavernous sinus syndrome

1 Trauma
2 Vascular:
    (a) posterior communicating artery aneurysm
    (b) intracavernous carotid artery
    (c) cavernous sinus thrombosis
    (d) carotico-cavernous fistula
3 Neoplasia:
    (a) intracranial tumours
    (b) nasopharyngeal tumours
    (c) metastases
4 Infection:
    (a) sinusitis
    (b) tuberculosis
5 Other inflammation: Wegener's granulomatosis.

Structures found in the cavernous sinus

1 Third, fourth and sixth cranial nerves
2 Ophthalmic branch of the fifth cranial nerve
3 Sympathetic carotid plexus
4 Intracavernous carotid artery.

Functions of the seventh (facial) nerve

1 Motor nerves to muscles of facial expression
2 Chorda tympani to anterior two-thirds of tongue
3 Taste from palate (nerve of pterygoid canal)
4 Parasympathetic fibres to parotid, submandibular and sublingual glands
5 Supplies stapedius muscle in the ear.

Causes of facial nerve palsy

1 Stroke
2 Multiple sclerosis
3 Otitis media
4 Brainstem tumour
5 Diabetes
6 Bell's palsy
7 Ramsay Hunt syndrome (herpes zoster infection)
8 Neurosarcoidosis
9 Acoustic neuroma
10 Lyme disease (borreliosis)
11 Cholesteatoma
12 Guillain–Barré syndrome.

Causes of bilateral facial nerve palsy

1 Myasthenia gravis
2 Bilateral Bell's palsies
3 Sarcoidosis
4 Guillain–Barré syndrome
5 Lyme disease
6 Mikulicz' syndrome (parotid infiltration).

Testing the eighth (vertibulocochlear) nerve

Rinne's test

1 Normal ear – air conduction greater than bone conduction
2 Nerve deafness – air conduction greater than bone conduction
3 Middle ear conduction defect – air conduction less than bone conduction.

Weber's test

A tuning fork is held to the middle of forehead. If sound is heard to one side there is either middle ear deafness on that side, or the opposing ear has nerve deafness.

Causes of deafness

Conduction

1 Ear wax
2 Middle ear infection
3 Otosclerosis.

Sensorineural

1 Acoustic neuroma
2 Ménière's disease
3 Paget's disease
4 Multiple sclerosis
5 CVA
6 Glioma
7 Head trauma
8 Drugs – aminoglycosides, furosemide (frusemide), lead
9 Congenital:
   (a) maternal infections
   (b) part of a congenital syndrome.

Causes of vertigo

Central (brainstem)

1 Multiple sclerosis
2 Space-occupying lesion, e.g. glioma

3 Vascular disease
4 Acute vestibular neuronitis
5 Hypoglycaemia
6 Alcohol
7 Drugs.

Peripheral (labyrinthine)

1 Trauma
2 Ménière's disease
3 Viral infection
4 Internal auditory artery occlusion
5 Chronic otitis media.

Acoustic neuroma

1 Eighth cranial nerve
2 Benign
3 Causes cerebellopontine angle syndrome
4 Treat by surgical removal.

MOVEMENT DISORDERS

Causes of ataxia

1 Vascular:
  (a) cerebellar/brainstem haemorrhage
  (b) cerebellar/brainstem infarct
  (c) arteriovenous malformation
2 Alcohol:
  (a) Wernicke's encephalopathy
  (b) chronic cerebellar degeneration
3 Autoimmune:
  (a) Miller Fisher syndrome
  (b) paraneoplastic cerebellar degeneration
  (c) paraneoplastic sensory neuropathy
  (d) Sjögren's disease
4 Multiple sclerosis
5 Neurodegenerative disease:
  (a) idiopathic late-onset cerebellar ataxia

(b) multiple system atrophy
6 Inherited:
  (a) spinocerebellar ataxia types 1–12 (autosomal dominant)
  (b) dentatorubropallidomysian atrophy (autosomal dominant)
  (c) hereditary motor and sensory neuropathy (Roussy–Levy variant)
  (d) Friedreich's ataxia (autosomal recessive)
  (e) ataxia telangiectasia (autosomal recessive)
  (f) ataxia with vitamin E deficiency (autosomal recessive)
  (g) mitochondrial disorders (maternal inheritance, sporadic)
  (h) ataxia may be a feature of numerous other inborn errors of metabolism
7 Infective:
  (a) encephalitis (varicella)
  (b) abscess
  (c) tuberculoma
  (d) CJD
  (e) syphilis (tabes dorsalis)
8 Drugs: lithium, phenytoins, mercury, cytarabine, pyridoxine, vincristine, paclitaxel
9 Developmental:
  (a) Arnold–Chiari malformation
  (b) Dandy–Walker syndrome
10 Tumours:
  (a) any primary intracranial neoplasm, including:
    (i) medulloblastoma
    (ii) pilocytic astrocytoma
    (iii) haemangioblastoma
  (b) metastases
11 Metabolic: vitamin B_{12} deficiency → subacute combined degeneration of the cord.

Benign essential tremor

1 Affects hands
2 Autosomal dominant
3 Worse with stress
4 Improves with alcohol
5 Treat with propanolol.

Causes of myoclonus

1 Physiological (falling asleep)
2 Liver failure
3 Renal failure
4 Alzheimer's disease
5 CJD
6 Drug-induced, e.g. amitriptyline
7 Gaucher's disease
8 Following cerebral anoxia (cardiac arrest)
9 Juvenile myoclonic epilepsy.

Causes of chorea

1 Huntington's disease
2 Syndenham's chorea (rheumatic)
3 Polycythaemia rubra vera
4 SLE
5 Thryrotoxicosis
6 Drugs:
    (a) OCP
    (b) phenytoin
    (c) neuroleptics (dopamine-blocking)
7 Pregnancy (chorea gravidarum)
8 Neuroacanthocytosis
9 Wilson's disease
10 Cerebellar degeneration
11 Hemiballismus
12 Paroxysmal choreoathetosis.

Huntington's disease

1 Autosomal dominant (chromosome 4)
2 Chorea
3 Cognitive decline
4 Positive family history
5 Neuroleptics used to relieve chorea.

Parkinsonism

Triad of:

1 Resting tremor
2 Bradykinesia
3 Rigidity.

Causes

1 Idiopathic Parkinson's disease
2 Drug-induced Parkinsonism
3 Normal-pressure hydrocephalus
4 Diffuse Lewy body disease
5 Progressive supranuclear palsy (PSP)
6 Dementia pugilistica – caused by chronic head injury, e.g. from boxing
7 Postencephalitic
8 Depression
9 'Parkinson's plus' syndromes
10 Multiple system atrophy, e.g. Shy–Drager syndrome
11 Toxins (narcotics, MPTP, carbon monoxide, manganese).

MUSCULAR DISORDERS

Duchenne muscular dystrophy

1 X-linked, 1 in 3500 male births
2 Xp21 region – codes of the absent dystrophin protein
3 Delay in reaching motor milestones
4 Affected muscles:
   (a) girdles
   (b) axial muscles
   (c) proximal limbs, particularly the legs
5 Pseudohypertrophy of calf muscles
6 Hyperkaemia
7 Ability to walk lost at around 12 years
8 Death by respiratory/cardiac failure in the 20s or early 30s.

Myotonic dystrophy (dystrophia myotonica)

1 Myotonic facies
2 Myotonia: unable to relax muscles following contraction, e.g. grip
3 Progressive muscular weakness and wasting, starting distally

4 Bilateral ptosis
5 Facial muscle weakness
6 Sternomastoid wasting
7 Cataracts
8 Insulin resistance   DM
9 Cardiac conduction defects
10 Bulbar weakness
11 Respiratory muscle weakness
12 Frontal balding
13 Mental retardation (in severe cases)
14 Testicular/ovarian atrophy.

Myasthenia gravis

1 Antibodies to acetylcholine receptors
2 Postsynaptic membrane of neuromuscular junction
3 Complement-mediated destruction of receptors.

Symptoms and signs

1 Ptosis
2 Ophthalmoplegia
3 Dysarthria
4 Fatiguable weakness of striated muscle
5 Respiratory muscle involvement is life threatening
6 Bulbar symptoms and nasal regurgitation
7 Head drooping if there is weakness of neck musculature.

Investigations

1 Acetycholine receptor antibodies (in around 90%)
2 Electromyography (EMG) – decreasing muscle action potential with
   repetitive motor nerve stimulation
3 Tensilon test – intravenous edrophonium, assesses immediate and
   short-acting effect of anticholinesterases
4 CT thorax – ? associated thymoma
5 Thyroid function – 10% have co-existent thyrotoxicosis.

Treatment

1 Pyridostigmine (cholinesterase inhibition)

2 Thymectomy
3 Steroids
4 Cyclophosphamide, ciclosporin (immunosuppression)
5 Plasmapheresis
6 Intravenous immunoglobulins.

Prognosis

1 Lifelong therapy required
2 Most controlled with few or no symptoms
3 Mortality slightly increased – associated with:
   (a) increased age
   (b) severe disease
   (c) presence of thymoma.

Eaton–Lambert myasthenic syndrome

1 Clinical features:
   (a) fatiguability
   (b) hyporeflexia
   (c) autonomic symptoms (micturition difficulty, dry mouth, constipation, impotence)
2 Ophthalmoplegia and ptosis *not* present
3 Reflexes return after exercise
4 EMG shows increasing response with repetitive nerve stimulation
5 Paraneoplastic syndrome, most common with small cell carcinoma of the lung
6 May occur without neoplasia.

Multiple sclerosis (MS)

Cell-mediated autoimmune disease associated with immune activity against myelin (demyelination).
Four subtypes:
1 Relapsing/remitting disease: 80–85% of patients
2 Secondary progressive disease: 30–50% of patients with relapsing/remitting form
3 Primary progressive disease: 10–15%, deterioration from onset
4 Progressive-relapsing disease: superimposed relapses.

NEUROLOGY

Symptoms

1 Weakness (40%)
2 Optic neuritis (22%)
3 Paraethesiae (21%)
4 Diplopia (12%)
5 Disturbance of micturition (5%)
6 Vertigo (5%).

Diagnosis

1 CNS lesions disseminated in time and place (anatomically)
2 Diagnosis not possible at the time of the first neurological event
3 Symptom patterns occur.

Investigations

1 MRI scan
2 Delayed visual-evoked response potentials
3 Oligoclonal bands in CSF (not in serum, non-specific).

Management

1 Intravenous methylprednisolone for acute attacks
2 Interferon-β – reduces frequency and severity of relapses
3 Antispasmodic, e.g. baclofen/tizanidine
4 Oxybutynin (anticholinergic) for urinary incontinence.

Prognosis

1 33% proceed to disabling paraparesis
2 25% incontinent or require catheterisation
3 15% are confined to a wheelchair
4 15% – severe cerebellar dysfunction
5 10% remain minimally disabled ten years after onset ('benign' MS)
6 75% are alive 35 years after diagnosis.

HEADACHE

Causes of chronic recurrent headaches

1 Tension headache
2 Classic or common migraine
3 Cluster headache
4 Headache due to increased intracranial pressure.

Migraine

1 Preceded by visual aura
2 Unilateral
3 Throbbing
4 Nausea
5 Photophobia
6 May rarely result in stroke
7 Neurological signs (reversible)
8 Vascular in origin – exact cause unsure.

Specific treatment

1 During an attack:
   (a) ergotamine
   (b) sumatriptan
2 Propylactic:
   (a) propranolol
   (b) pizotifen
   (c) amitriptyline
   (d) methysergide.

Cluster headache

1 Clusters may last days or weeks
2 More common in men.
3 Clinical features:
   (a) unilateral pain
   (b) lacrimation
   (c) retro-orbital pain
   (d) nasal rhinitis
4 Treatment:

(a) ergotamine, sumatriptan, oxygen, for acute attack
(b) lithium for prophylaxis.

NEUROLOGICAL INVESTIGATIONS

Normal cerebrospinal fluid (CSF) (see also page 247)

1 Pressure: 60–150 mm of H_2O (8–12 cm saline) with the patient lying down
2 Protein 0.2–0.4 g/litre
3 Cell count:
     (a) zero red cells
     (b) < 5/mm³ white cells
4 Glucose: over two-thirds of blood glucose (2.8–4.0 mmol/litre).

Complications of lumbar puncture

1 Herniation of brain or spinal cord
2 Headache
3 Meningitis or epidural abscess
4 Intrathecal bleeding
5 Damage to or infection of intervertebral disc
6 Intraspinal dermoid cyst.

Causes of raised CSF pressure

1 Space-occupying lesions or acute brain swelling
2 High venous pressure, e.g. dural sinus thrombosis
3 Benign intracranial hypertension
4 Hydrocephalus.

Increased CSF protein concentration

Raised

1 Bacterial meningitis
2 Viral encephalitis
3 Cerebral abscess
4 Multiple sclerosis
5 Cerebral tumours (primary and metastases)

6 Cerebral infarction
7 Subdural haematoma
8 Dural sinus thrombosis.

Markedly raised

2–6 g/litre.
1 Guillain–Barré syndrome
2 Spinal block (secondary to tumour)
3 TB meningitis
4 Fungal meningitis.

White cells in CSF

1 Polymorphs: bacterial meningitis
2 Lymphocytes:
  (a) viral encephalitis/meningitis
  (b) partially treated bacterial meningitis
  (c) CNS vasculitis
  (d) HIV-associated
  (e) lymphoma
  (f) leukaemia
  (g) Lyme disease
  (h) SLE
  (i) Behçet's syndrome
  (j) polio
  (k) multiple sclerosis
  (l) dural sinus thrombosis
  (m) stroke.

Reduced or absent CSF glucose

1 Bacterial meningitis
2 TB meningitis
3 Malignant meningitis, i.e. atypical – fungal, mumps
4 Herpes simplex encephalitis
5 Subarachnoid haemorrhage.

Oligoclonal bands in CSF

1 Multiple sclerosis

2 Adrenoleukodystrophy
3 Neurosarcoidosis
4 Neurosyphilis
5 Neuro-AIDS
6 CNS lymphoma
7 Subacute sclerosing panencephalitis
8 Guillain–Barré syndrome
9 Subarachnoid haemorrhage
10 Neuro-Lyme disease.

Intracranial calcification on head CT/skull X-ray

1 Craniopharyngioma
2 Meningioma
3 Tuberculoma
4 Oligodendroglioma
5 Pineal gland
6 Tuberose sclerosis
7 Sturge–Weber syndrome
8 Toxoplasmosis
9 Hypoparathyroidism
10 Aneurysm.

Electroencephalography (EEG)

The diagnosis of epilepsy

1 Interictal epileptiform discharges (IEDs)
2 Focal or generalised IEDs starting focally seen in partial epilepsy
3 Generalised symmetrical IEDs in generalised epilepsy
4 3-Hz spike- and wave-complexes in absence seizures.

Other characteristic EEG patterns

1 Creutzfeldt–Jakob disease: short-interval periodic discharges
2 Subacute sclerosing panencephalitis: long-internval periodic discharges
3 Encephalitis: diffuse slow-wave activity.

Electromyography (EMG)

1 Myasthenia gravis: decreased response to repetitive stimulation

2 Eaton–Lambert syndrome: increased response to repetitive
stimulation
3 Myotonia: 'dive-bomber' discharge
4 Polymyositis; fibrillation potentials; low-amplitude polyphasic motor
unit action potentials (MUAP)
5 Motor neurone disease: fibrillation (degeneration); shape of MUAPs
changes (re-innervation).

Ophthalmology

EYE SIGNS IN MEDICAL DISORDERS

Table 42

Sign	Disorder
Lisch nodules	Neurofibromatosis
Brushfield's spots	Down's syndrome
Kayser–Fleischer rings	Wilson's disease
Band keratopathy	Hypercalcaemia
	Chronic uveitis
Bitot's spots	Vitamin A deficiency
Corneal arcus	Hypercholesterolaemia (types 2a and 2b)
	Old age
Blue sclera	Osteogenesis imperfecta
	Pseudoxanthoma elasticum
	Ehlers–Danlos syndrome
	Marfan's syndrome
	Hyperthyroidism
Angioid streaks	Pseudoxanthoma elasticum
	Ehlers–Danlos syndrome
	Paget's disease
	Sickle cell disease
Corneal calcification	Sarcoidosis
	Hyperparathyroidism
	Chronic renal failure
	Vitamin D abuse

Diabetic eye disease

Diabetic eye disease is the most common cause of blindness in patients aged 30–60 years.

1 *Background retinopathy:*
   (a) visual acuity unaffected
   (b) microaneurysms

(c) haemorrhages
(d) hard exudates
2 *Preproliferative retinopathy:*
(a) cotton-wool spots
(b) dilatation and beading of retinal veins
(c) intraretinal microvascular abnormalities
3 *Proliferative retinopathy* (more common in type 1 diabetics):
(a) neovascularisation
(b) treated cases will have panretinal laser burns
4 *Advanced diabetic eye disease:*
(a) vitreous haemorrhage
(b) tractional retinal detachment
(c) rubeotic glaucoma
5 *Maculopathy* (more common in type 2 diabetics):
(a) oedema and exudates
(b) macular stars (multiple exudates)
(c) loss of central vision (peripheral vision spared).

Criteria for referral to an ophthalmologist

1 Preproliferative retinopathy
2 Proliferative retinopathy
3 Maculopathy
4 Advanced diabetic eye disease.

Treatment

1 Good diabetic control
2 Treatment of hypertension
3 Stopping smoking
4 Treatment of hypercholesterolaemia
5 Regular fundal examination
6 Focal retinal photocoagulation
7 Panretinal photocoagulation.

HYPERTENSIVE RETINOPATHY

Grade 1 – silver wiring of retinal arteries
Grade 2 – grade 1 plus arteriovenous nipping and focal arteriolar
attenuation

Grade 3 – grade 2 plus haemorrhages, hard exudates and cotton-wool spots

Grade 4 – grade 3 plus papilloedema.

CAUSES OF COTTON-WOOL SPOTS

1 Diabetes mellitus
2 Hypertension
3 Vasculitis
4 HIV retinopathy
5 Septicaemia
6 Haemoglobinopathy
7 Radiation retinopathy
8 Myeloproliferative disorders
9 Fat emboli.

THYROID EYE DISEASE

Signs

NO SPECS:
1 **N** o signs or symptoms may be evident
2 **O** nly upper-lid retraction and stare
3 **S** oft tissue swelling
4 **P** roptosis
5 **E** xtraocular muscle involvement (lymphocytic infiltration of inferior and medial recti)
6 **C** orneal involvement (keratoconjunctivitis)
7 **S** ight loss due to optic nerve damage (optic neuropathy).

Management

Severe disease

1 High-dose steroids
2 Orbital irradiation
3 Plasma exchange
4 Orbital decompression.

Mild to moderate disease

1 Symptomatic treatment
2 Artificial tears
3 Prisms for diplopia
4 Tarsorrhaphy.

CAUSES OF PAPILLOEDEMA

1 Raised intracranial pressure, due to:
  (a) space-occupying lesions:
    (i) tumour
    (ii) haematoma
    (iii) abscess
  (b) meningitis/encephalitis
  (c) subarachnoid haemorrhage
  (d) cerebral oedema
  (e) aqueduct stenosis
  (f) AV malformation
2 Hypertensive retinopathy
3 Benign intracranial hypertension
4 Metabolic causes:
  (a) CO_2 retention
  (b) vitamin A intoxication
  (c) lead poisoning
  (d) Graves' disease
  (e) hypoparathyroidism
5 Oral contraceptives
6 Tetracyclines
7 Central retinal vein thrombosis
8 Cavernous sinus thrombosis
9 Severe anaemia
10 Polycythaemia rubra vera
11 Paget's disease
12 Guillain–Barré syndrome
13 Hurler's syndrome.

CAUSES OF OPTIC ATROPHY

1 Congenital:
   (a) Leber's optic atrophy
   (b) DIDMOAD syndrome (diabetes insipidus, diabetes mellitus, optic atrophy and deafness)
   (c) Friedreich's ataxia
2 Multiple sclerosis
3 Compression of the optic nerve:
   (a) tumour (craniopharygioma, pituitary adenoma)
   (b) aneurysm
   (c) orbital cellulitis
4 Glaucoma
5 Chronic papilloedema
6 Ischaemia:
   (a) retinal artery occlusion
   (b) temporal arteritis
   (c) tabes dorsalis
7 Diabetes mellitus
8 Nutritional deficiency:
   (a) vitamins B_1, B_2, B_6, B_{12}
   (b) alcohol-tobacco amblyopia
9 Toxic:
   (a) methanol
   (b) alcohol
   (c) arsenic
   (d) lead
10 Dysthyroid eye disease
11 Toxoplasmosis
12 Syphilis
13 Paget's disease
14 Retinitis pigmentosa
15 Drugs:
   (a) ethambutol
   (b) isoniazid
   (c) digitalis
   (d) chlorpropamide.

OPTIC NEURITIS

1 Inflammation of the optic nerve
2 Unilateral reduction of acuity over hours to days
3 Colours (particularly red) appear less intense
4 Painful eye movements
5 Relative afferent pupillary defect present
6 Optic disc swollen
7 Recovery occurs over 2–6 weeks
8 45–80% develop MS over the next 15 years
9 Treat with high-dose methylprednisolone for three days – reduces risk of developing MS over the next two years.

CAUSES OF CHOROIDORETINITIS

1 CMV
2 Toxoplasmosis
3 Toxocariasis
4 AIDS
5 Sarcoidosis
6 TB
7 Syphilis
8 Behçet's syndrome
9 Trauma
10 Idiopathic.

RETINAL VEIN THROMBOSIS

1 Central retinal vein occlusion or branch retinal vein occlusion
2 Presents with loss of vision or reduced acuity
3 Can be treated with panretinal photocoagulation
4 *Fundoscopy* may reveal:
    (a) multiple retinal haemorrhages
    (b) retinal venous dilatation
    (c) cotton-wool spots
    (d) neovascularisation
5 *Causes:*

(a) hypertension
(b) diabetes mellitus
(c) glaucoma
(d) hyperviscosity (myeloma and macroglobulinaemia)
(e) polycythaemia
(f) vasculitides.

RETINAL ARTERY OCCLUSION

1 Presents with sudden painless loss of vision
2 Afferent pupillary defect
3 Leads to pale fundus
4 Cherry-red spot may be present for up to ten days
5 *Causes:*
   (a) embolus (AF, carotid artery stenosis)
   (b) thrombosis
   (c) vasculitides (particularly giant-cell arteritis)
   (d) increased orbital pressure
   (e) sickle cell disease
   (f) syphilis
   (g) spasm (cocaine, retinal migraine).

CAUSES OF CATARACT

1 Congenital:
   (a) autosomal dominant
   (b) maternal infection:
       (i) rubella
       (ii) CMV
       (iii) toxoplasmosis
       (iv) HSV
       (v) varicella zoster
   (c) metabolic:
       (i) galactosaemia
       (ii) galactokinase deficiency
       (iii) hypocalcaemia
       (iv) hypoglycaemia

    (d) chromosomal abnormalities
      (i) Down's syndrome
      (ii) Turner's syndrome
2 Senile
3 UV light
4 Drugs:
    (a) steroids
    (b) chlorpromazine
    (c) chloroquine
    (d) busulfan
    (e) gold
    (f) amiodarone
5 Ocular conditions:
    (a) uveitis
    (b) high myopia
6 Metabolic:
    (a) diabetes mellitus
    (b) Cushing's syndrome
    (c) hypoglycaemia
    (d) Wilson's disease
    (e) hypoparathyroidism
    (f) Fabry's disease
7 Trauma
8 Radiation
9 Myotonic dystrophy
10 Retinitis pigmentosa.

CAUSES OF LENS DISLOCATION

1 Trauma
2 Marfan's syndrome (upwards)
3 Homocystinuria (downwards)
4 Uveal tumours.

CAUSES OF UVEITIS

1 Idiopathic

2 Ankylosing spondylitis
3 Reiter's syndrome
4 Psoriatic disease
5 Inflammatory bowel disease
6 Sarcoidosis
7 Behçet's syndrome
8 Juvenile chronic arthritis
9 Malignancy:
  (a) non-Hodgkin's lymphoma
  (b) retinoblastoma
  (c) ocular melanoma
10 Trauma
11 Infections:
  (a) TB
  (b) syphilis
  (c) HSV
  (d) VZV
  (e) toxoplasmosis
  (f) toxocariasis
  (g) AIDS
12 leprosy
13 brucellosis
14 histoplasmosis
15 onchocerciasis.

CAUSES OF SCLERITIS

1 Rheumatoid arthritis
2 PAN
3 SLE
4 Wegener's granulomatosis
5 Relapsing polychondritis
6 Dermatomyositis
7 Behçet's syndrome
8 Ankylosing spondylitis
9 Sarcoidosis
10 Inflammatory bowel disease
11 Gout

12 Infections:
   (a) VZV
   (b) HSV
   (c) TB
   (d) syphilis
   (e) toxoplasmosis
   (f) *Pseudomonas*
   (g) *Streptococcus*
   (h) *Staphylococcus*
13 Trauma
14 Chemicals.

RETINITIS PIGMENTOSA

1 Degenerative disease of the retina
2 AR, AD or X-linked inheritance
3 Mainly affects rods (cones may be involved late in the disease)
4 Presents with night blindness
5 Peripheral vision lost first (tunnel vision)
6 Most patients are registered blind by the age of 40 years
7 Characterised by perivascular 'bone spicule pigmentation', arteriolar narrowing and optic atrophy
8 *Associations:*
   (a) Laurence–Moon and Biedl–Bardet syndromes
   (b) Bassen–Kornzweig syndrome (abetalipoproteinaemia)
   (c) Refsum's disease
   (d) Kearns–Sayre syndrome
   (e) Usher's disease
   (f) Friedreich's ataxia.

RETINOBLASTOMA

1 Malignant tumour of the retina
2 Usually affects children under the age of three years
3 Bilateral in 30%
4 The retinoblastoma gene (*RB*) is a tumour suppressor gene present in everyone

5 Those with retinoblastoma inherit one abnormal retinoblastoma gene and develop the tumour when the other (normal) gene spontaneously mutates
6 *Presentation:*
  (a) white pupil
  (b) squint
  (c) inflammation
  (d) loss of red reflex
7 Increased incidence of osteosarcoma
8 Treatment is by enucleation.

GLAUCOMA

Acute (closed-angle) glaucoma

1 Uniocular
2 Caused by blockage of the drainage of aqueous from the anterior chamber via the canal of Schlemm
3 Most likely to occur when the pupil is semi-dilated in the dark
4 *Presentation:*
  (a) red eye
  (b) pain
  (c) vomiting
  (d) reduced vision
  (e) dilated pupil
  (f) hazy cornea
5 *Treatment:*
  (a) acetazolamide (reduces the formation of aqueous)
  (b) pilocarpine (constricts the pupil, opening the canal)
  (c) peripheral iridectomy.

Chronic (open-angle) glaucoma

1 Increased intraocular pressure ($> 21\,\text{mmHg}$)
2 Insidious asymptomatic onset
3 Leads to cupping of the optic disc and nerve damage
4 Arcuate scotomas near the blind spot
5 *Risk factors:*
  (a) family history

  (b) Afro-Caribbean origin
  (c) diabetes mellitus
  (d) myopia
  (e) thyroid eye disease
6 *Treatment* (aim is to reduce the intraocular pressure):
  (a) timolol drops (reduces secretion of aqueous)
  (b) pilocarpine drops
  (c) acetazolamide
  (d) latanoprost (prostaglandin $F_{2\alpha}$ analogue that increases outflow of aqueous)
  (e) laser trabeculoplasty
  (f) trabeculectomy.

PTOSIS

Causes of unilateral ptosis

1 Congenital
2 Idiopathic
3 Third nerve palsy
4 Horner's syndrome
5 Myasthenia gravis
6 Lid tumour.

Causes of bilateral ptosis

1 Myasthenia gravis
2 Dystrophia myotonica
3 Ocular myopathy
4 Mitochondrial dystrophy
5 Tabes dorsalis
6 Bilateral Horner's (syringomyelia).

Psychiatry

SCHIZOPHRENIA

1 Incidence equal in all social classes
2 Prevalence 1%, male and female equal, greatest in lower social class
3 Onset age 15–45 years (males younger than females)
4 Some genetic predisposition
5 10% commit suicide, especially in the early stages.

First-rank symptoms

Described by Kurt Schneider.
1 Auditory hallucinations:
    (a) third-person voices discussing the patient
    (b) audible thoughts/echo
    (c) commentary on actions
2 Passivity:
    (a) thought insertion, withdrawal or broadcast
    (b) feeling of thoughts, actions being under external control
3 Delusions.

Good prognostic factors

1 Acute onset
2 Precipitating stressful event
3 No family history of schizophrenia
4 Older age of onset
5 No previous episodes
6 Normal intelligence
7 Preponderance of affective symptoms
8 No loss of emotion
9 Family history of depression.

Treatment

1 Antipsychotics: useful for positive symptoms, i.e. delusions, hallucinations. Older drugs cause extrapyramidal side-effects
2 Electroconvulsive therapy (ECT) for stupor
3 Cognitive behavioural therapy.

BIPOLAR AFFECTIVE DISORDER

1 Lifetime prevalence of 1% with slight female preponderance
2 Symptoms mainly of increased mood
3 Usually preceded or followed by depression.

Features

1 Elevated, elated mood
2 Irritability
3 Insomnia
4 Loss of inhibitions
5 Increased appetite but weight loss
6 Increased libido
7 Flight of ideas
8 Pressure of speech
9 Poor attention span
10 Delusions of grandeur.

Treatment is with lithium to stabilise mood.

DEPRESSION

1 Lifetime incidence – up to 20%
2 Twice as common in females
3 Old classification: endogenous *versus* reactive.

Biological symptoms

1 Anhedonia
2 Sleep disorder (early-morning wakening)
3 Loss of appetite

4 Weight loss
5 Decreased libido
6 Retardation, loss of concentration
7 Diurnal variation (worse in the morning).

Depression in the elderly

1 More common in females with previous history and physical illness
2 17% remain chronically depressed; 30% die within six years
3 Poorer prognosis if associated with physical illness, organic brain disease or onset after the age of 70 years.

Response to antidepressant drugs

The following features are associated with a better response to antidepressants:
1 Normal premorbid personality
2 Presence of biological features
3 Previous history of bipolar disorder.

EATING DISORDERS

1 More common in higher social classes
2 5% of patients are male.

Anorexia nervosa

Diagnosis

1 Self-induced loss of > 15% of body weight
2 Morbid fear and avoidance of 'fattening' foods
3 Distorted ideas of and overestimation of body size
4 Overuse/abuse of exercise, purgatives
5 Amenorrhoea for more than three months.

Bulimia nervosa

1 Binge eating and vomiting
2 Preoccupation with eating
3 May be overweight.

Features associated with poor outcome

1 Long duration
2 Older at onset
3 Lower weight
4 Vomiting
5 Bulimia
6 Poor parental relationship.

Mortality is 25% untreated; 5% treated. Only 35% recover fully.

Medical complications

1 Bradycardia and hypotension
2 Arrhythmias
3 Low FSH/LH/oestrogens and amenorrhoea
4 Osteoporosis and fractures
5 Proximal myopathy, cramps and tetany
6 Pancytopenia and hypoplastic bone marrow
7 Hypothermia and dehydration
8 Electrolyte disturbances (especially hypokalaemia)
9 Reversible brain atrophy and seizures
10 Hypercholesterolaemia
11 Dental decay
12 GI erosions and ulceration
13 Nephropathy.

OBSESSIVE COMPULSIVE DISORDER

Obsessions: recurrent persistent ideas which the patient recognises as abnormal,but resistance to which causes upset.
Compulsions: thoughts about carrying out an action, triggered by obsessions.
1 Slight female preponderance
2 30% have associated depression
3 25% with depression get obsessions
4 Associated with anorexia nervosa, schizophrenia and organic brain disease
5 *Treatment:*
   (a) serotonin reuptake inhibitors (TCAs, SSRIs)
   (b) antipsychotics if antidepressants are ineffective

(c) cognitive behavioural therapy
(d) surgery may be effective.

SYMPTOMS OF ANXIETY DISORDERS

1 Wide spectrum of physical and mental symptoms
2 Anxious thoughts
3 Hyperventilation and breathlessness
4 Palpitations
5 Chest pain
6 Headaches
7 Tingling
8 Nausea
9 Loose bowel motions
10 Urinary frequency.

SUICIDE AND PARASUICIDE

Risk factors for suicide

1 Male
2 Young or late middle age
3 Social classes I or V
4 Chronic illness
5 Chronic pain
6 Physical handicap
7 Psychiatric illness
8 Depression
9 Alcoholism
10 Unemployment
11 Farmers and doctors.

Risk factors for deliberate self-harm

1 Female
2 Age < 35 years
3 Social classes IV and V
4 History of depression
5 May have antisocial personality.

ALCOHOL

Acute alcohol withdrawal (delerium tremens)

1 Tremor
2 Visual hallucinations
3 Acute confusion
4 Insomnia
5 Agitation
6 Pyrexia
7 Onset after 72 hours without alcohol
8 May have an associated infection
9 Electrolyte deficiencies are often seen (potassium, magnesium)
10 5% mortality.

Features of alcohol dependence syndrome (cage)

1 May have tried to **c**ut down alcohol
2 **A**nger at criticism of drinking
3 **G**uilt at drinking
4 **E**arly-morning drinking
5 Drinking usually is in a fixed pattern
6 Repeated absenteeism from work
7 Awareness of compulsion to drink
8 Increased tolerance to alcohol
9 Frequent symptoms of withdrawal.

Wernicke's encephalopathy (see also page 312)

1 Caused by acute thiamine deficiency
2 *Features:*
   (a) gross confusion
   (b) ataxia
   (c) nystagmus
   (d) abducens and conjugate gaze palsies
3 Microvascular lesions in third and fourth ventricles, periaqueductal grey matter, mamillary bodies, brainstem and cerebellum
4 Cortex usually spared
5 Treatment with intravenous thiamine
6 80% develop Korsakoff's syndrome.

Note: non-alcohol-related causes of Wernicke's include:

1 Pregnancy
2 Repeated persistent vomiting
3 Carcinoma of the stomach
4 Dietary deficiency.

Korsakoff's syndrome

1 Usually a consequence of Wernicke's
2 Markedly impaired short-term recall
3 Anterograde amnesia
4 Variable retrograde amnesia
5 Registration normal
6 Lack of insight
7 Confabulation common.

May also follow carbon monoxide poisoning or herpes simplex encephalopathy.

ORGANIC BRAIN DISEASE

Acute confusional state (acute organic brain syndrome)

1 Causes may be intra- or extracranial
2 Usually reversible
3 May be due to disordered blood–brain barrier.

Intracranial causes

1 Head injury
2 CNS infection (encephalitis, meningitis)
3 Epilepsy
4 Space-occupying lesion
5 Intracranial bleed (subarachnoid, intracerebral, subdural)
6 Cerebrovascular disease.

Extracranial causes

1 Infections (e.g. UTI, chest)
2 Toxic:
    (a) alcohol
    (b) drugs – prescribed or illicit

3 Endocrine:
   (a) thyroid disease
   (b) diabetes
   (c) adrenal disease especially Cushing's
4 Electrolyte disorder (sodium, calcium)
5 Metabolic:
   (a) hypoglycaemia
   (b) uraemia
   (c) hepatic encephalopathy
6 Systemic (SLE).

DEMENTIA (see also pages 302–305)

Dementia

Defined as progressive, global impairment of cognitive function with clear consciousness.

Alzheimer's disease

1 Affects 5% of over 65s, 20% of over 80s
2 Onset mainly 70–90 years
3 Affects more females than males (due to increased life expectancy)
4 Insidious onset, diffuse cognitive impairment, early loss of insight
5 Classical microscopic appearance of neurofibrillary tangles, senile plaques and glial proliferation
6 Characteristic loss of cholinergic neurones
7 Death usually occurs 2–5 years after diagnosis.

Multi-infarct disease

1 Less common than Alzheimer's disease
2 Affects men more than women
3 Age of onset 60–80 years
4 Acute onset, variable cognitive impairment, insight spared
5 Associated with previous CVA/TIA and risk factors for these
6 Death occurs 4–5 years from diagnosis.

Pick's disease

1 Age of onset 50–60 years

2 Twice as common in females
3 Atrophy of frontal lobes
4 Pick cells are pathognomonic.

Other causes of dementia

1 Huntington's chorea
2 Neurosyphilis
3 Creutzfeld–Jakob disease
4 Multiple sclerosis
5 Normal-pressure hydrocephalus.

DRUGS AND PSYCHIATRY

Benzodiazepines

1 Short-term anxiolytics
2 Withdrawal characterised by anxiety, restlessness, hyperstimulation and increased REM sleep
3 Withdrawal: commonest in short-acting drugs (may occur within hours); may not be seen until 7–10 days in long-acting drugs
4 Withdrawal lasts 7–10 days.

Antipsychotics

1 Useful for positive symptoms of schizophrenia
2 Sedative action more immediate than antipsychotic effect
3 Phenothiazines (chlorpromazine, thioridazine) cause marked extrapyramidal side-effects
4 Butyrophenones (haloperidol) – marked anticholinergic and antiadrenergic side-effects.

Electroconvulsive therapy

1 Indicated for treatment of marked depressive illness with biological symptoms, especially stupor
2 *Side-effects:*
   (a) headache
   (b) impaired short-term memory
   (c) confusion

(d) fractures and dislocations
3 *Contraindications:*
   (a) raised intracranial pressure (absolute)
   (b) recent MI/CVA
   (c) cardiac arrhythmia
   (d) brain tumour (relative).

Respiratory Medicine

PHYSIOLOGY

Pulmonary blood flow is approximately 5,000 ml/minute.
Alveolar ventilation is approximately 5,250 ml/minute.

Respiratory function tests

Total lung capacity (TLC)

1 6–7 litres in the normal adult
2 Measured by body plethysmography or helium dilution technique.

Tidal volume (TV)

1 Volume of normal resting breath
2 Approximately 500 ml in the normal adult.

Vital capacity (VC)

1 End of forced inspiration to the end of forced expiration
2 75% of TLC
3 Decreases with age
4 Depends on height, age, sex and ethnic origin.

Forced vital capacity (FVC)

1 Volume of maximal forceful expiration after maximal inspiration
2 Reduced in restrictive disorders
3 May be normal or increased in obstructive disorders.

Forced expiratory volume₁ (FEV₁)

1 Volume expired in one second of maximal expiration after maximal inspiration
2 Normal is 75–80% of FVC
3 Variables are the same as for VC
4 Reduced in obstructive airways disease; a marker of severity of disease.

Peak expiratory flow rate (PEFR)

1 Flow rate of first 0.01 second of maximal expiration
2 Variables as for VC
3 Only measures calibre of medium and large airways.

Compliance

A measure of the distensibility of lung tissue and airways.
1 ↑ Emphysema
2 ↓ Fibrosis, pulmonary oedema.

Blood gases

Oxygenation of haemoglobin

1 Hb is changed from ferric to ferrous form
2 Fetal haemoglobin (HbF) has greater affinity for O_2
3 Partial pressure of O_2 and saturation (SaO_2) follows oxygen dissociation curve
4 Increased affinity for O_2 represents shift of curve to the RIGHT.

Causes of increased O_2 affinity

1 ↑Temperature
2 ↑ H^+, i.e. ↓ pH
3 ↑ P_aCO_2
4 ↑ 2,3 DPG (adaptation to altitude, chronic anaemia).

Note that these are all things which happen in working muscle.

Gas transfer factor

1 Measure of gas diffusion across alveolar membrane into capillaries
2 Depends on blood volume, blood flow, surface area of membrane and

distribution of ventilation
3 Measured by diffusion of carbon monoxide (TLco)
4 The transfer coefficient Kco is the above, corrected for lung volume.

Causes of decreased transfer factor

1 COPD
2 Interstitial lung disease
3 Pulmonary embolus
4 Pneumonia
5 Pulmonary oedema
6 Pulmonary hypertension
7 Pneumonectomy.

Causes of increased transfer factor

1 Pulmonary haemorrhage
2 Exercise
3 Polycythaemia
4 Asthma (when well)
5 Left–right shunt.

RESPIRATORY FAILURE

Type I

Hypoxaemia, $PO_2 < 8\,kPa$ (60 mmHg) with normal PCO_2.

Causes

1 Early stages of severe asthma
2 Emphysema
3 Pneumonia
4 Pulmonary embolus
5 Pulmonary oedema
6 Interstitial lung disease
7 ARDS.

Treatment

Treated by increasing inspired concentration of oxygen (FIO_2).

Type II

Hypoxaemia with CO_2 retention, $P_{CO_2} > 6.7$ kPa (50 mmHg).

Causes

1 COPD
2 Late stages of severe asthma
3 Neurological disorders (Guillain–Barré, MND, MS)
4 Muscular disease (myasthenia gravis, muscular dystrophy)
5 Chest wall disease (kyphoscoliosis, ankylosing spondylitis, surgery)
6 Drugs (opioids).

Treatment

1 Usually treated with mechanical ventilatory support
2 Respiratory stimulants (doxepram) of limited use.

ASTHMA

Chronic asthma

1 Incidence 20% in children, 15% in adults
2 Chronic inflammatory disorder with variable airflow obstruction
3 Combination of genetic predisposition and environmental atopy
4 Mediated by IgE, prostaglandin-derived growth factor (PDGF) and
  interleukins.

Cells involved

1 Mast cells
2 Macrophages
3 Epithelial cells
4 Eosinophils.

Pulmonary function tests

1 >25% variation in PEFR
2 ↓ FEV_1
3 ↓ FEV_1/FVC ratio
4 PEFR and FEV_1 ↑ post-bronchodilator
5 ↑ Lung volume.

Trigger factors for acute attacks

1 Exposure to allergen (pollen, house-dust mite, cat and dog dander)
2 Exercise
3 Drugs (NSAIDs and aspirin, beta-blockers)
4 Infection
5 Oesophageal reflux
6 Smoke
7 Non-compliance with medication.

Acute asthma

Causes 1500 deaths per year in the UK.

Markers of severe acute asthma

1 Difficulty speaking
2 Tachycardia >110 b.p.m.
3 Pulsus paradoxus
4 Respiratory rate >30/minute
5 PEFR <33% of best/predicted
6 Silent chest
7 Hypoxia
8 Normal or raised PCO_2.

Management

1 High-flow O_2
2 Nebulised bronchodilators
3 Steroids
4 ? Antibiotics
5 Intravenous aminophylline or salbutamol
6 ? Ventilation.

Exercise-induced asthma

1 Characteristically occurs 5–10 minutes after exercise
2 Lasts less than one hour
3 Worse in cold air
4 Prevented by beta-agonist pre-exercise
5 Exercise in following four hours causes fewer problems.

Causes of occupational asthma

1 Isocyanates (paint, plastics, insulation)
2 Flour
3 Grain dusts
4 Soldering flux (colophony fumes)
5 Epoxy resins
6 Proteolytic enzymes (detergent manufacture)
7 Platinum salts
8 Laboratory animals.

DISEASES CAUSED BY *ASPERGILLUS FUMIGATUS*

Allergic bronchopulmonary aspergillosis

1 Seen in 1–2% of asthmatics
2 Nearly always seen in association with asthma, but not invariably
3 Type I and type III hypersensitivity reaction
4 IgE and IgG antibodies to *Aspergillus fumigatus*
5 Associated with eosinophilia and positive precipitins
6 Perihilar infiltrate, lobar collapse, upper-lobe fibrosis and proximal bronchiectasis on CXR
7 May see fungal hyphae in sputum/lavage fluid
8 Aspergillosis may become invasive in immunocompromised patients – treat with amphotericin.

Aspergilloma

1 Damaged lung colonised with ball of fungus (mycetoma)
2 May be seen on CXR (cavitate) and CT
3 Complicated by haemorrhage
4 Treat with surgery/radiotherapy.

CHRONIC OBSTRUCTIVE PULMONARY DISEASE (COPD)

1 Chronic progressive airflow obstruction, mainly non-reversible
2 Biggest aetiological factor is smoking

3 Marked morbidity/mortality
4 FEV$_1$/FVC ratio $<75\%$; FEV$_1$ $<80\%$ of predicted values.

Long-term oxygen therapy (LTOT)

1 Proven to increase three-year survival by 50% in eligible patients
2 Need to raise Po$_2$ to >60 mmHg for over 15 hours per day
3 Strict criteria for prescription (all of below):
   (a) arterial blood gases must be measured on two occasions, three weeks apart, when the patient is free from exacerbation
   (b) Po$_2$ <7.3 kPa (55 mmHg), or 7.3–8.0 kPa (55–60 mmHg) with evidence of cor pulmonale
   (c) Pco$_2$ normal or raised
   (d) FEV$_1$ <1.5 litres
   (e) non-smoker
   (f) Po$_2$ on oxygen should rise to >8 kPa (60 mmHg) without a significant rise in Pco$_2$.

Alpha-1-antitrypsin deficiency

1 Autosomal dominant
2 Most severe is the PiZZ phenotype
3 Presents in the third to fourth decades
4 Marked panlobular emphysema in basal lung areas
5 Worse in smokers
6 Associated with liver cirrhosis.

BRONCHIECTASIS

Irreversible dilatation of small airways. Obstructive spirometry due to plugging by secretions. Appearances may be saccular, atelectatic or follicular.

Causes

Congenital

1 Selective IgA deficiency
2 Kartagener's syndrome (ciliary dyskinesis associated with infertility, dextracardia and situs inversus)

3 Primary immotile cilia syndrome
4 X-linked hypogammaglobulinaemia.

Acquired

1 Childhood pneumonia, pertussis, measles
2 Post-TB
3 Allergic bronchopulmonary aspergillosis
4 Distal to obstructed bronchus (foreign body, tumour)
5 Associated with pulmonary fibrosis and sarcoid
6 Idiopathic.

Features

1 Chronic production of purulent sputum
2 Exertional breathlessness
3 Clubbing
4 Early/mid-inspiratory crepitations
5 CXR shows thickened bronchial walls and ring shadows
6 Obstructive or restrictive spirometry
7 High-resolution CT usually diagnostic.

CYSTIC FIBROSIS

1 Autosomal recessive
2 One in 25 adults are carriers
3 Incidence is 1 in 2000 live births
4 Gene on long arm of chromosome 7 codes for cystic fibrosis transmembrane regulator protein (CFTR)
5 Over 300 mutations – commonest is deletion of three bases called ΔF_{508} (68% cases)
6 Defect of chloride and water transport across the epithelial cell membrane
7 Diagnosis is by sweat test: sodium and chloride concentrations >60 mmol/l
8 Life expectancy now reaching the forties.

Respiratory features

1 Obstruction of small airways with thick mucus due to reduced chloride

secretion and increased sodium resorption
2 Colonisation with *Staphylococcus aureus, Haemophilus influenzae* and *Pseudomonas aeruginosa*
3 *Burkholderia cepacia* increasingly important, highly transmissible
4 Chronic infection and inflammation with bronchiectasis
5 Respiratory failure in late stages
6 Treat with antibiotics, acutely and prophylactically, oral ± nebulised
7 Transplantation

Gastrointestinal features

1 Pancreatic insufficiency in 80% (steatorrhoea, vitamin deficiency) – oral pancreatic supplements are given
2 Meconium ileus in infancy; small-bowel obstruction in adults
3 Chronic liver disease seen due to biliary tree obstruction (<5%)
4 Gallstones
5 Pancreatitis.

Other features

1 Diabetes (>30% of patients in late teens)
2 Nasal polyps (30%)
3 Pneumothorax (5%)
4 Infertility (almost all men)
5 Osteoporosis.

PULMONARY FIBROSIS

Causes

1 Upper-lobe fibrosis:
   (a) sarcoidosis
   (b) TB
   (c) pneumoconiosis
   (d) silicosis
   (e) histiocytosis
   (f) ankylosing spondylitis
   (g) ABPA
2 Lower-lobe fibrosis:
   (a) bronchiectasis

    (b) asbestosis
    (c) CFA
    (d) RA
    (e) drugs
    (f) systemic sclerosis
    (g) radiation
3 Drug-induced fibrosis:
    (a) amiodarone
    (b) methotrexate
    (c) azathioprine
    (d) nitrofurantoin
    (e) bleomycin
    (f) busulfan
    (g) chlorambucil.

Cryptogenic fibrosing alveolitis (CFA)

1 More common in men
2 *Clinical features:*
    (a) dry cough
    (b) breathlessness
    (c) clubbing
    (d) cyanosis
    (e) fine late-inspiratory crepitations
3 Diagnosed by high resolution CT scanning, restrictive spirometry, bibasal interstitial shadowing on CXR, type I respiratory failure
4 Circulating ANF or RF in 25%.

Extrinsic allergic alveolitis

IgG-mediated type III and type IV hypersensitivity reaction to inhaled particles. Causes pneumonitis.
1 *Farmer's lung:* caused by thermophilic actinomyces (*Micropolyspora faeni* and *Thermoactinomyces vulgaris*) in mouldy hay
2 *Bird fanciers' lung:* seen in keepers of pigeons and budgerigars. Due to keratin in faeces and feather bloom
3 *Bagassosis:* due to *Thermoactinomyces sacchari* in sugar cane
4 *Ventilation pneumonitis:* caused by thermophilic actinomyces in humidification systems of air-conditioned buildings

5 *Malt workers' lung:* caused by *Aspergillus clavatus*
6 *Mushroom workers' lung:* caused by thermophilic actinomyces.

Clinical features

1 Fever, cough and breathlessness four to nine hours after exposure. No wheeze. Settles in 48 hours
2 CXR may be normal; may show nodular shadows and hazy infiltrate
3 Chronic disease causes irreversible fibrosis and restrictive spirometry
4 Serum precipitins helpful in diagnosis
5 No eosinophilia
6 Bronchoalveolar lavage shows lymphocytosis and normal to low CD4/CD8 count
7 Transbronchial biopsy may show mononuclear infiltrates and granulomata
8 Treatment is avoidance of the precipitant and steroids in acute illness (though no improvement in outcome in chronic disease).

OCCUPATIONAL LUNG DISEASE

Coal-workers' pneumoconiosis (CWP)

1 Occurs 10–20 years after exposure
2 Small particles retained in alveoli and small bronchioles
3 Small rounded opacities in the lung fields on CXR
4 Background CWP may go on to progressive massive fibrosis (PMF)
5 Large opacities > 10 mm on CXR in PMR. Usually upper lobe. May cavitiate
6 Mixed obstructive/restrictive spirometry pattern
7 Compensatable (only if there are CXR changes)
8 Caplan's syndrome – multiple lung nodules in patient with rheumatoid arthritis and CWP. Usually peripheral.

Silicosis

1 Inhaled silicon dioxide in rock-face miners, quarry workers, engineers and sandblasters
2 Subacute phase occurs within a few months of exposure – and dry cough
3 Progresses to upper-lobe nodule formation

4 Late stages – restrictive lung disease
5 Previously showed a marked increase in the incidence of TB
6 Only treatment is transplant
7 Compensatable.

Berylliosis

1 Acute beryllium fume inhalation causes alveolitis
2 Chronic exposure causes sarcoid-like illness
3 Non-caseating granulomata and fibrous lymph nodes
4 CXR – bilateral hilar lymphadenopathy and diffuse fine nodules
5 Interstitial fibrosis develops.

Byssinosis

1 Inhalation of cotton dust, hemp or flax
2 Symptoms worse on Monday morning – improves over the week
3 Symptoms occur one to six hours after exposure
4 Cough, breathlessness and wheeze
5 More common in smokers
6 CXR normal
7 Compensatable.

Diseases caused by exposure to asbestos

Pleural plaques and thickening

1 Occur 20 or more years after exposure
2 Plaques on parietal pleura
3 Usually asymptomatic
4 May progress to diffuse, confluent thickening, causing exertional breathlessness
5 Restrictive spirometry, Kco normal.

Asbestosis

1 Occurs 20 years or more after exposure
2 Lower lobe fibrosis
3 Dry cough, exertional breathlessness, lower-zone crepitations and clubbing
4 CXR shows irregular shadowing, with ring and honeycomb patterns in more advanced disease

5 Restrictive spirometry and low Kco
6 Associated with an increased incidence of lung cancer
7 Compensatable.

Mesothelioma

1 85% of cases are due to asbestos
2 See below, in section on lung cancer.

GRANULOMATOUS LUNG DISEASE

Sarcoidosis

1 A multisystem disease
2 Cause unknown
3 Mainly affects young adults
4 Prevalence 25/100,000
5 Three times more common in Afro-Caribbeans
6 Characteristic lesion is a non-caseating granuloma
7 Associated with HLA-A1, HLA-B8 and HLA-DR3.

Clinical features (see also page 92)

1 There may be no respiratory symptoms
2 Dry cough, fever, breathlessness, weight loss
3 Examination often shows nothing abnormal, occasional clubbing
4 Bilateral hilar lymphadenopathy and erythema nodosum are almost
   diagnostic
5 May progress to irreversible fibrosis – upper and mid-zones usually
   affected
6 May rarely see upper airway involvement with obstruction and
   discharge.

Chest X-ray classification

Stage 0   Normal CXR
Stage 1   Bilateral hilar lymphadenopathy (BHL)
Stage 2   BHL and pulmonary infiltrates
Stage 3   Diffuse infiltration.

Diagnosis

1 Transbronchial biopsy diagnostic in 85% of stage 1 cases
2 Raised calcium and ACE levels
3 Kveim test positive in 75% – no longer recommended
4 High resolution CT scanning.

Extrapulmonary manifestations

1 Liver (40–70%): subclinical granuloma infiltration
2 Cardiac (30–70%):
   (a) cardiac muscle problems
   (b) arrhythmias
3 Skin (25%):
   (a) erythema nodosum
   (b) nodules
   (c) plaques
   (d) lupus pernio
4 Eyes (25%): anterior uveitis
5 Splenomegaly (25%)
6 Neurological (5%):
   (a) meningitis
   (b) hydrocephalus
   (c) space-occupying lesions
   (d) cranial nerve palsy
   (e) spinal cord involvement
   (f) may affect posterior pituitary
7 Bone:
   (a) cysts (small bones of the hands and feet)
   (b) arthritis (Löfgens syndrome – triad of BHL, polyarthritis and erythema nodosum).

Treatment

1 May not need any treatment
2 Steroids
3 Azathioprine, methotrexate
4 Hydroxychloroquine
5 Thalidomide.

Prognosis

Stage 1 – 80% spontaneous remission
Stage 2 – 50% spontaneous remission
Stage 3 – 30% spontaneous remission.

Poor prognostic factors

1 Stage 3
2 Age >40 years
3 Symptoms >6 months
4 No erythema nodosum
5 More than three systems involved
6 Splenomegaly.

Histiocytosis X

1 Diffuse infiltrative eosinophilic granulomata
2 Usually young males
3 Strongly associated with smoking.

CONNECTIVE TISSUE DISEASE AND THE LUNG

Lung involvement is seen in:
1 Rheumatoid arthritis (nodules, fibrosis, bronchiectasis, Caplan's syndrome, effusion)
2 SLE (fibrosis, shrinking lung syndrome)
3 Systemic sclerosis (fibrosis, bronchiectasis).

Causes of pulmonary vasculitis

1 Ulcerative colitis
2 Multiple PE
3 Giant cell arteritis
4 Takayasu's disease
5 Behçet's disease.

Churg–Strauss syndrome: necrotising pulmonary vasculitis, granulomata and eosinophilic infiltrates. pANCA positive, 50%.

LUNG CANCER

The commonest cancer in the West.

Causes

1 Smoking (95%)
2 Industrial (asbestos, arsenic, benzoyl chloride, aluminium salts)
3 Atmospheric (pollution, passive smoking)
4 Associated with CFA and systemic sclerosis.

Cell types

1 Squamous (52%): arise in the central airway
2 Small cell (21%): central airway, rapidly growing and metastasise early.
3 Adenocarcinoma (11%): may be peripheral
4 Large cell (10%)
5 Bronchiolar-alveolar cell (6%).

Complications
Physical/metastatic

1 Pleural effusion
2 Dysphagia
3 SVC obstruction
4 Recurrent laryngeal nerve palsy (hoarseness)
5 Phrenic nerve palsy (raised hemidiaphragm)
6 Pericarditis and effusion
7 Spontaneous pneumothorax.

Non-metastatic

1 SIADH (small cell)
2 Ectopic ACTH syndrome (small cell)
3 Hypercalcaemia (metastases, squamous cell mediated by PTHrP)
4 Gynaecomastia (large cell)
5 Clubbing (commonest in non-small cell)
6 Eaton–Lambert syndrome (small cell): proximal myopathy and reduced tendon reflexes

7 Hypertrophic pulmonary osteoarthropathy (squamous cell): arthritis, clubbing and periostitis. Commonly affects long bones.

Treatment

1 Surgery for non-small cell. Only 20% are operable. Five-year survival post-surgery only 25%
2 Palliative/radical radiotherapy
3 Chemotherapy (small cell): improves survival.

Contraindications to surgery

1 Small-cell type
2 Local invasion (laryngeal nerve, oesophagus etc.)
3 Distant metastasis, including mediastinal nodes
4 Bloody pleural effusion
5 FEV_1 <1.5 litres
6 Tumour <1.5 cm from carina.

Prognosis

1 Median survival for small-cell tumours is 14 months in limited disease, 10 months in extensive disease
2 Five-year survival for non-small-cell tumours is 10%.

Mesothelioma

1 One thousand cases per year in the UK
2 More common in men
3 85% due to asbestos exposure
4 Blue (crocidolite) > brown (amosite) > white (crysotile)
5 Presents 20–50 years after exposure
6 No cure
7 Median survival 16 months.

Bronchial carcinoid

1 Accounts for 1% of lung tumours
2 Cherry-red ball in bronchial tree
3 Occasionally associated with carcinoid syndrome (1–2%)
4 Histology similar to small-cell carcinoma
5 Five-year survival 90%.

PNEUMONIA (see also pages 238–239)

Community-acquired pneumonia

1 Incidence is 3 per 1000 per year
2 Causal organisms:
   (a) *Streptococcus pneumoniae* (60–75%)
   (b) atypical (5–18%):
      (i) *Mycoplasma pneumoniae*
      (ii) *Legionella*
      (iii) *Chlamydia psittaci* and *Chlamydia pneumoniae*
   (c) *H. influenzae* (5%)
   (d) *S. aureus*
   (e) viruses (influenza, varicella).

Mycoplasma *pneumonia*

1 Affects young adults
2 Epidemics every 3–4 years
3 Long prodromal phase
4 May be associated with cold agglutinins.

Legionella *pneumonia*

1 Contaminated air-conditioning, showers, water cooling systems
2 There is often underlying lung disease
3 Jaundice may occur
4 WCC may be normal, with lymphopenia
5 SIADH and low sodium
6 Abnormal LFTs in 50%
7 Neurological signs and symptoms are common.

Staphylococcus *pneumonia*

1 May complicate influenza
2 Common in intravenous drug abusers
3 Associated with lung abscess and empyema.

Hospital-acquired pneumonia

1 Organisms:

(a) *S. aureus*
(b) Gram-negative organisms (*Klebsiella*, *Proteus*, *E. coli*, *Pseudomonas*)
(c) anaerobes
2 Treatment is with third-generation cephalosporins.

Pneumocystis carinii pneumonia (PCP)

1 Organism is an atypical fungus
2 Commonest in immunocompromised patients
3 Symptoms of dry cough, fever and breathlessness
4 CXR may be normal, or show diffuse perihilar shadowing
5 Diagnosis by bronchoscopy, washings and silver stain or PCR
6 Treatment is with Septrin® ± pentamidine, and steroids if $Po_2 < 9.3\,kPa$ (70 mmHg)
7 Mortality 5%.

Causes of eosinophilic pneumonia

1 Allergic aspergillosis
2 Drugs (sulfasalazine, nitrofurantoin, imipramine)
3 Other infections
4 Parasites
5 Smoke inhalation.

Markers of severity in pneumonia (BTS guidelines 2 or more = severe)

Age >65

1 Diastolic BP <60 mmHg
2 Serum urea >7 mmol/l
3 Respiratory rate >30 per minute
4 Confusion.

TUBERCULOSIS

Incidence is increasing.

At-risk groups

1 Immigrants from endemic areas
2 Alcoholics

3 HIV-positive
4 Homeless
5 Low income.

Primary TB

1 May be entirely asymptomatic
2 Infection in a person with no immunity
3 Ghon focus develops in the lung
4 Bacilli are transported through lymphatics
5 Infection is then arrested
6 Tuberculin tests become positive after this
7 May cause mild cough, wheeze and erythema nodosum.

Post-primary TB

This occurs on reactivation of disseminated dormant organisms.

Miliary TB

Widespread haematological spread of bacilli.

Symptoms

1 Night sweats
2 Weight loss
3 Cough
4 Haemoptysis
5 Pleural effusion
6 Meningitis.

Diagnosis

1 CXR (upper-lobe shadowing, loss of volume, cavitation)
2 Sputum examination for acid-alcohol-fast bacilli (AAFBs)
3 Early morning urine for AAFBs
4 Lymph node biopsy
5 Bone marrow aspirate
6 Bronchoscopy and lavage
7 Culture takes at least six weeks
8 PCR available.

Treatment of TB

1 In HIV-negative Caucasians with no previous treatment or contact, treat with triple therapy – rifampicin, isoniazid and pyrazinamide
2 Others – add ethambutol
3 Triple/quadruple therapy for two months, then rifampicin/isoniazid for a further four months
4 Rifampicin, isoniazid, pyrazinamide are all bactericidal, ethambutol is bacteristatic
5 Compliance is very important
6 Side-effects common:
  (a) rifampicin:
    (i) hepatitis
    (ii) nausea
    (iii) pink/orange urine
    (iv) enzyme inducer
    (v) may precipitate Addisonian crisis
  (b) isoniazid:
    (i) hepatitis
    (ii) peripheral neuropathy (cover with pyridoxine)
  (c) pyrazinamide:
    (i) hepatitis
    (ii) rash
    (iii) gout
  (d) ethambutol:
    (i) optic neuritis
    (ii) renal dysfunction.

Multidrug-resistant TB – 2% of all cases.

Atypical TB organisms

Clinically and radiologically indistinguishable from *Mycobacterium tuberculosis* infection – cause 10% of infections:
1 *Mycobacterium malmoensae*
2 *Mycobacterium kansasii*
3 *Mycobacterium xenopi*
4 *Mycobacterium avium* intracellulare.

OBSTRUCTIVE SLEEP APNOEA

1 Incidence 1–2%, middle-aged men
2 Ten or more episodes of apnoea of at least ten seconds' duration per hour
3 Occurs in REM sleep
4 Airway obstruction at base of tongue/soft palate due to loss of muscle tone
5 Symptoms of daytime somnolence, snoring and headaches
6 Causes are obesity (80%), acromegaly, hypothyroidism, alcohol and Marfan's syndrome
7 Diagnosis – Epworth sleep score and overnight pulse oximetry
8 Treatment – weight loss and nasal CPAP.

PLEURAL EFFUSION

1 *Transudate* (protein <30 g/l):
   (a) cardiac failure
   (b) cirrhosis
   (c) hypoalbuminaemia
   (d) nephrotic syndrome
   (e) hypothyroidism
   (f) dialysis
2 *Exudate* (protein >30 g/l):
   (a) parapneumonic
   (b) TB
   (c) subphrenic abscess
   (d) PE
   (e) pancreatitis (amylase in fluid)
   (f) asbestos
   (g) rheumatoid disease (RF in fluid)
   (h) SLE
   (i) malignancy
3 Fluid glucose low in:
   (a) RA
   (b) TB
   (c) malignancy
   (d) empyema.

CAUSES OF HAEMOPTYSIS

1 Lung cancer
2 TB
3 PE
4 Bronchiectasis
5 Aspergilloma
6 Pulmonary abscess
7 Farmer's lung
8 Wegener's granulomatosis
9 Goodpasture's syndrome
10 PAN
11 Haemosiderosis
12 Endometriosis.

CAVITATION ON CXR

1 Bullae
2 Pneumonias (*Klebsiella*, staphylococcal, anaerobic)
3 TB
4 Abscess
5 Tumour (squamous cell, secondaries)
6 PE
7 Pneumoconiotic nodule
8 Rheumatoid nodule
9 Wegener's granulomatosis
10 Churg–Strauss syndrome
11 Honeycomb lung (systemic sclerosis)
12 Progressive massive fibrosis.

CALCIFICATION ON CXR

1 Lung:
  (a) TB
  (b) carcinoma
  (c) chickenpox
  (d) sarcoid

    (e) asbestos exposure
    (f) silicosis
    (g) pneumoconiosis
    (h) hydatid disease
    (i) schistosomiasis
2 Pleura:
    (a) asbestos exposure
    (b) empyema
    (c) haemothorax
    (d) TB
    (e) recurrent pneumothorax
3 Lymph nodes:
    (a) TB
    (b) carcinoid
    (c) silicosis
4 Other sites:
    (a) pericardium
    (b) heart valves
    (c) aorta.

Rheumatology

COMMON CAUSES OF ACUTE MONOARTHRITIS

1. Acute septic arthritis
2. Gout
3. Pseudogout
4. Trauma
5. Seronegative spondyloarthritides
6. Rheumatoid arthritis (RA)
7. Haemarthrosis
8. Foreign body synovitis
9. Neuropathic arthropathy
10. Local malignant deposit
11. Avascular necrosis.

CAUSES OF ACUTE POLYARTHRITIS

1. RA
2. Generalised osteoarthritis (OA)
3. Viral infections:
   (a) rubella (also rubella vaccine)
   (b) mumps
   (c) parvovirus
   (d) coxsackievirus
   (e) varicella
   (f) echovirus
   (g) adenovirus
   (h) arbovirus (including dengue fever)
   (i) hepatitis A, B and C
   (j) EBV
   (k) CMV
   (l) HSV
   (m) rhinovirus type 7
   (n) HIV

4 Reiter's syndrome
5 Seronegative arthritides
6 Gonococcal arthritis
7 Adult and childhood-onset Still's disease
8 Rheumatic fever
9 SLE
10 TB
11 Gout (10% are polyarthropathy)
12 Pyrophosphate arthropathy
13 Serum sickness
14 Acute sarcoidosis
15 Familial Mediterranean fever
16 HSP
17 Type 2 hyperlipoproteinaemia
18 Leukaemia
19 Paraneoplastic syndromes
20 Polymyalgia rheumatica
21 Drug allergies.

CHARACTERISTICS OF SYNOVIAL FLUID IN HEALTH AND DISEASE

Table 43

Source	Colour	Culture	Clarity	Viscosity	WCC($\times 10^6$/l)
Normal	Yellow	Negative	Clear	High	<200
OA	Yellow	Negative	Clear	High	<200
RA	Yellow/green	Negative	Clear/turbid	Low	3,000–50,000
Bacterial arthritis	Purulent	Positive	Turbid	Low	50,000–100,000
Gout	Yellow/white	Negative	Clear	Low	100–150,000
Pseudogout	Yellow/white	Negative	Clear/ bloodstained	Low	50–75,000

BACTERIA ASSOCIATED WITH SPECIFIC ARTHRITIDES

Septic arthritis

1 *Staphylococcus aureus*
2 *Streptococcus pyogenes*
3 *Staphylococcus epidermidis*
4 *Streptococcus pneumoniae*
5 *Mycobacterium tuberculosis*
6 *Neisseria gonorrhoeae*
7 *Haemophilus influenzae*
8 *Salmonella* spp.
9 *Bacteroides fragilis*
10 *Enterococcus faecium*
11 *Enterococcus faecalis*
12 *Escherichia coli*
13 *Klebsiella pneumoniae*
14 *Proteus mirabilis*
15 *Pseudomonas aeruginosa.*

Osteomyelitis

1 *Staphylococcus aureus*
2 *Bacteroides fragilis*
3 Enterobacteriaceae
4 *Mycobacterium tuberculosis*
5 Non-group A streptococci
6 *Peptostreptococcus anaerobius*
7 *Provotella melaninogenica*
8 *Pseudomonas aeruginosa.*

CRYSTAL-RELATED ARTHROPATHIES

Gout

Negatively birefringent needle-shaped crystals of monosodium urate. The biochemical abnormality in gout is hyperuricaemia.

Causes of hyperuricaemia

Increased production

1 Increased purine synthesis:
   (a) idiopathic
   (b) hypoxanthine-guanine-phosphoribosyl transferase deficiency (Lesch–Nyhan syndrome – X-linked)
   (c) phosphoribosyl-pyrophosphate synthetase overactivity (X-linked)
   (d) ribose-5-phosphate overproduction
   (e) AMP-deaminase deficiency
2 Increased turnover of preformed purines:
   (a) lymphoproliferative and myeloproliferative disorders
   (b) cytotoxic drugs
   (c) carcinomatosis
   (d) secondary polycythaemia
   (e) chronic haemolytic anaemias
   (f) severe exfoliative psoriasis
   (g) Gaucher's disease.

Decreased excretion

1 Reduction in fractional urate clearance:
   (a) idiopathic
   (b) chronic renal failure
   (c) familial juvenile gouty nephropathy (AD)
   (d) increased levels of organic acids (alcohol, starvation, exercise, ketoacidosis)
   (e) hypertension
   (f) hyperparathyroidism
   (g) hypothyroidism
   (h) Down's syndrome
   (i) lead nephropathy
   (j) sarcoidosis
   (k) Bartter's syndrome
2 Drug administration
   (a) diuretics (thiazides and loop diuretics)
   (b) salicylates (low-dose)
   (c) pyrazinamide
   (d) ethambutol
   (e) nicotinic acid

(f) ciclosporin.

Events provoking gouty arthritis

1 Trauma
2 Unusual physical exercise
3 Surgery
4 Severe systemic illness
5 Severe dieting
6 Dietary excess
7 Alcohol
8 Drugs (above + allopurinol and probenecid).

Pyrophosphate arthropathy (pseudogout)

Positively birefringent rhomboid crystals of calcium pyrophosphate leads to chondrocalcinosis.

Causes

1 Older age
2 OA
3 Familial
4 Diabetes mellitus
5 Hyperparathyroidism
6 Haemochromatosis
7 Hypophosphataemia
8 Hypomagnesaemia
9 Hypothyroidism
10 X-linked hypophosphataemic rickets
11 Familial hypocalciuric hypercalcaemia
12 Wilson's disease
13 Ochronosis
14 Acromegaly
15 Lead poisoning.

RHEUMATOID ARTHRITIS

Revised American College of Rheumatology criteria for the classification of rheumatoid arthritis (1987)

A diagnosis of rheumatoid arthritis can be made if at least four of the following features are present:
1 Morning stiffness (>1 hour) for >6 weeks
2 Arthritis of three or more joint areas for >6 weeks
3 Arthritis of the hand joints for >6 weeks
4 Symmetrical arthritis
5 Rheumatoid nodules
6 Serum rheumatoid factor
7 Radiographic changes.

Joint involvement in RA

Symmetrical polyarthropathy affecting the following joints:

MCP	90%
PIP	90%
MTP	90%
Wrists	80%
Knees	80%
Ankle/subtalar	80%
Shoulder	60%
Hip	50%
Elbow	50%
Acromioclavicular	50%
Cervical spine	40%
TMJ	30%
Sternoclavicular	30%
Cricoarytenoid	10%

Extra-articular features of RA

Non-organ specific

1 Weight loss
2 Malaise
3 Fever
4 Lymphadenopathy

5 Rheumatoid nodules
6 Felty's syndrome
7 Amyloidosis
8 Increased susceptibility to infections
9 Osteoporosis.

Organ specific

Vasculitic

1 Splinter haemorrhages
2 Distal gangrene
3 Nail fold infarcts
4 Cutaneous ulceration
5 'Palpable purpura'
6 Peripheral neuropathy
7 Organ vasculitis (e.g. mesenteric)
8 Pulmonary.

Cardiac

1 Pericarditis and effusion
2 Constrictive pericarditis
3 Endocarditis and valvular heart disease
4 Myocarditis.

Pulmonary

1 Pleurisy
2 Pleural effusion
3 Interstitial fibrosis
4 Nodular lung disease
5 Bronchiolitis obliterans
6 Airways obstruction
7 Caplan's syndrome (nodules and progressive massive fibrosis in coal
   workers)
8 Cricoarytenitis.

Renal

1 Drug-induced:
   (a) second-line agents (gold and penicillamine) – membranous
        glomerulonephritis

(b) NSAIDs – interstitial nephritis and minimal change glomerulonephritis
(c) renal papillary necrosis secondary to analgesic abuse
2 Amyloidosis
3 Renal tubular acidosis (RTA) type 1.

Neurological

1 Compressive neuropathies, e.g. carpal tunnel syndrome
2 Mononeuritis multiplex (a result of vasculitis)
3 Cervical myelopathies.

Ocular

1 Episcleritis
2 Scleritis
3 Scleromalacia perforans
4 Sjögren's syndrome
5 Extraocular paralysis (resulting from mononeuritis multiplex)
6 Cataracts (steroid therapy).

Other features

1 Palmar erythema
2 Pyoderma gangrenosum.

Factors associated with poorer prognosis in RA

1 Insidious polyarticular onset
2 Female patients
3 Extra-articular manifestations
4 Functional disability at one year after the start of the disease
5 Substantially raised concentration of rheumatoid factors
6 Presence of HLA-DR4
7 Family history of RA
8 Radiographic evidence of erosions within one year of disease onset.

Laboratory findings in RA

1 Anaemia – normochromic or hypochromic, normocytic
2 Thrombocytosis

3 ↑ ESR
4 ↑ CRP
5 ↑ Ferritin
6 ↓ Iron concentration
7 ↓ TIBC
8 ↑ Globulins
9 ↑ ALP
10 Rheumatoid factor.

Rheumatoid factor (RF)

1 IgM, IgG or IgA antibodies against the Fc component of IgG antibodies
2 Agglutination tests (latex) detect IgM RF (seropositive disease)
3 ELISA tests detect IgM and IgG RF
4 Found in 80% of patients with RA
5 Found in 5% of the general population (up to 25% in over 75s)
6 Role is unclear in the pathogenesis of RA
7 Extra-articular features are commoner in patients with high concentrates of RF
8 Positive RF is a poor guide to the severity of joint disease
9 RF is positive in other conditions (see below).

Causes of a positive RF

1 Connective tissue diseases (often high titre, > 1/160):
   (a) RA   80% (extra-articular 100%)
   (b) Sjögren's syndrome   75–100%
   (c) RA+ sicca syndrome   98%
   (d) SLE   20–40%
   (e) systemic sclerosis   5–10%
   (f) PAN   0–5%
   (g) dermatomyositis   0–5%
2 Chronic infections (usually low titre):
   (a) syphilis   10%
   (b) leprosy   50%
   (c) endocarditis 25%
   (d) TB   5–20%
3 Autoimmune liver diseases
4 Sarcoidosis
5 Mixed essential cryoglobulinaemia

6 Paraproteinaemias
7 Transplant recipients.

Causes of anaemia in RA

1 Anaemia of chronic disease
2 Iron deficiency – NSAIDs
3 Bone marrow suppression – gold, penicillamine, sulfasalazine and cytotoxics
4 Folate deficiency – sulfasalazine, methotrexate
5 Vitamin B_{12} deficiency – associated pernicious anaemia
6 Haemolysis – dapsone, sulfasalazine
7 Felty's syndrome.

Radiological features in RA

1 Soft-tissue swelling
2 Loss of joint space due to erosion of articular cartilage
3 Juxta-articular osteoporosis
4 Marginal bone erosions
5 Joint deformities.

Drug treatments for RA

Symptom-modifying drugs

1 Analgesics
2 NSAIDs.

Disease-modifying drugs

1 Antimalarials
2 Sulfasalazine
3 Gold
4 Penicillamine
5 Corticosteroids
6 Methotrexate
7 Azathioprine
8 Ciclosporin
9 Cyclophosphamide
10 Infliximab.

SERONEGATIVE SPONDYLOARTHRITIDES

Associated with HLA-B27, except Behçet's disease.
1 Ankylosing spondylitis
2 Psoriatic arthritis
3 Enteropathic arthritis:
   (a) Crohn's
   (b) UC
   (c) Whipple's disease
4 Reiter's syndrome/reactive arthritis
5 Behçet's disease (can also be classified as a vasculitis).

Comparison of seronegative spondyloarthritides and seropositive RA

Table 44

	Seronegative	Seropositive
Peripheral arthritis	Asymmetrical	Symmetrical
Spinal involvement	Ankylosis	Cervical subluxation
Cartilaginous joints	Commonly affected (SI joints)	Rarely affected
Tissue typing	HLA-B27	(HLA-DR4)
Eye	Anterior uveitis	Scleritis
	Conjunctivitis	Sicca syndrome
Skin	Psoriasis	Cutaneous nodules
	Keratoderma blenorrhagica	Vasculitis
	Mucosal ulceration	
	Erythema nodosum	
Heart	AR	Pericarditis
	Conduction defects	
Pulmonary	Chest-wall ankylosis	Nodules
	Apical fibrosis	Effusions
		Fibrosis
GI	Ulceration of small or large intestine	Drug-induced symptoms
GU	Urethritis	
	Genital ulceration	

Common features of seronegative spondyloarthritides

1 Negative RF
2 Asymmetrical inflammatory peripheral arthritis (oligoarthritis)
3 Radiological sacroiliitis
4 Spondylitis
5 Enthesitis
6 HLA-B27 association (96% in ankylosing spondylitis)
7 Anterior uveitis
8 Evidence of clinical overlap between diseases.

Associated diseases of the gut

1 Acute bacterial infection
2 Giardiasis and amoebiasis
3 UC/Crohn's disease
4 Whipple's disease
5 Coeliac disease
6 Jejunoileal bypass syndrome.

Ankylosing spondylitis

European Spondyloarthropathy Study Group diagnostic criteria for ankylosing spondylitis

Inflammatory spinal pain or synovitis plus any one of the following:
1 Positive family history
2 Psoriasis
3 Inflammatory bowel disease
4 Alternate buttock pain
5 Enthesopathy
6 Sacroiliitis.

Clinical features

The 'A' disease.
1 **A**rthritis
2 **A**tlano-axial subluxation
3 **A**nterior uveitis
4 **A**pical pulmonary fibrosis
5 **A**myloidosis
6 **A**ortic regurgitation

7 **A** ortitis
8 **A** –V conduction defects
9 Cauda equin**A** syndrome
10 Ig**A** nephropathy
11 **A** chilles tendonitis
12 Plantar f**A**sciitis.

Radiological features

1 SI joints:
    (a) irregular joint margins
    (b) subchondral erosion
    (c) sclerosis
    (d) fusion
2 Spine:
    (a) loss of lumbar lordosis
    (b) vertebral squaring
    (c) syndesmophyte formation (calcification of the annulus fibrosis)
    (d) bamboo spine (calcification in anterior and posterior spinal ligaments)
3 Peripheral joints: erosive arthropathy
4 Enthesopathies.

Reiter's syndrome/reactive arthritis

Triggers

1 *Chlamydia trachomatis*
2 *Campylobacter jejuni*
3 *Salmonella* spp.
4 *Shigella flexneri*
5 *Neisseria gonorrhoeae*
6 *Borrelia burgdorferi*
7 *Streptococcus pyogenes*
8 *Yersinia enterocolitica*
9 *Yersinia pseudotuberculosis.*

Clinical features

HLA-B27 80%.

Classic triad

1 Arthropathy
2 Conjunctivitis
3 Urethritis.

Other features

1 Sacroiliitis
2 Plantar fasciitis
3 Circinate balanitis
4 Keratoderma blennorrhagica
5 Anterior uveitis
6 Oral ulceration
7 Dystrophic nails
8 Fever
9 Pericarditis
10 Aortitis
11 Cardiac conduction defects
12 Pleurisy
13 Meningoencephalitis
14 Peripheral neuropathy.

Psoriatic arthropathy

Patterns of disease

1 Peripheral oligoarthritis or polyarthritis (60%)
2 Spondylitis (15%)
3 Distal interphalangeal disease (10%)
4 Rheumatoid type (10%)
5 Arthritis mutilans (5%).

Radiological features of psoriatic arthritis in peripheral joints

1 Relative lack of juxta-articular osteoporosis compared with RA
2 Periostitis and bony remodelling within the joints leading to 'pencil-in-cup' erosions
3 Osteolysis leading to complete dissolution of phalanges in some cases
4 Ankylosis.

Treatment for spondyloarthropathies

1 Physiotherapy
2 Local steroid injection
3 NSAIDs
4 Systemic steroids
5 Sulfasalazine
6 Methotrexate
7 Antibiotics (acute infections).

Behçet's disease

1 Oral ulceration
2 Genital ulceration
3 Uveitis
4 Phlebitis leading to thrombosis
5 Synovitis
6 Arthralgia/arthritis
7 Cutaneous vasculitis
8 Erythema nodosum
9 Meningoencephalitis
10 Large artery aneurysms
11 Discrete intestinal ulcers (bloody diarrhoea)
12 Pathergy (excessive erythema following skin prick)
13 Epididymitis.

CONNECTIVE TISSUE DISEASES

Systemic lupus erythematosus (SLE)

American College of Rheumatology revised criteria for the diagnosis of SLE (1982)

SLE is diagnosed if four or more of the following are present:
1 Malar rash
2 Discoid rash
3 Photosensitivity
4 Oral ulcers
5 Arthritis
6 Serositis (pleurisy, pericarditis)

  7 Renal disease (persistent proteinuria > 0.5 g/day, cellular casts)
  8 Neurological disorder (seizures, psychosis)
  9 Haematological disorder (haemolytic anaemia, leucopenia, lymphopenia, thrombocytopenia)
  10 Immunological disorder (LE cells, anti-ds DNA antibody, anti-Sm or false positive VDRL)
  11 Antinuclear antibody.

Clinical features

Constitutional symptoms

1 Fever
2 Fatigue
3 Anorexia
4 Nausea.

Mucocutaneous (81%)

1 Rash (malar, discoid, photosensitive)
2 Alopecia
3 Oral, nasal or vaginal ulcers
4 Raynaud's phenomenon (50%)
5 Livedo reticularis
6 Cutaneous vasculitis
7 Sjögren's syndrome
8 Purpura.

Musculoskeletal (95%)

1 Migratory asymmetrical non-erosive (Jaccoud's) arthritis
2 Myalgia
3 Myositis
4 Avascular necrosis of the femoral head.

Renal (53%)

1 Glomerulonephritis
2 Proteinuria
3 Nephrotic syndrome
4 Hypertension
5 End-stage renal failure (<5%)

6 Tubulointerstitial disease
7 Renal vasculitis.

Respiratory (48%)

1 Pleurisy
2 Recurrent pneumonitis
3 Shrinking lung syndrome
4 Cor pulmonale from pulmonary hypertension.

Cardiovascular (38%)

1 Pericarditis
2 Cardiomyopathy
3 Myocarditis
4 Coronary vasculitis – myocardial ischaemia
5 Libman–Sacks endocarditis.

CNS (59%)

1 Headaches
2 Migraine
3 Seizures
4 Chorea
5 Psychosis
6 Poor memory
7 CVA – vasculitis
8 Mononeuritis multiplex
9 Aseptic meningitis.

Haematological

1 Neutropenia
2 Lymphopenia
3 Thrombocytopenia
4 Lymphadenopathy
5 Splenomegaly
6 Hyposplenism
7 Antiphospholipid syndrome.

Gastrointestinal

1 Abdominal pain
2 Mesenteric vasculitis
3 Peptic ulcer disease (drugs)
4 Chronic active hepatitis.

Investigations

1 Normochromic normocytic anaemia with active disease
2 Leucopenia/lymphopenia
3 Raised ESR
4 Normal CRP (unless accompanied by serositis, synovitis or infection)
5 ANA positive in 95%
6 Raised immunoglobulins
7 Low C3 and C4
8 Antiphospholipid antibodies in 30–40%
9 Coombs positive haemolytic anaemia.

Patterns of staining of ANA

Table 45

Staining	Disease
Homogeneous	SLE
Speckled	MCTD, Sjögren's syndrome
Nucleolar	Scleroderma
Centromere	Limited systemic sclerosis (CREST)

Causes of a positive ANA

1 SLE (95%)
2 Sjögren's (80%)
3 Polymyositis/dermatomyositis (80%)
4 RA (30%)
5 Systemic sclerosis
6 CAH
7 Chronic infections
8 Malignancy
9 Old age.

Autoantibody associations with clinical syndromes in SLE

Table 46

Clinical syndrome	Autoantibody
Nephritis, photosensitivity, serositis	Anti-dsDNA
Photosensitivity	Anti-Ro/La
Neonatal lupus syndromes	Anti-Ro/La
Coagulopathy, thrombocytopenia, miscarriages, CNS syndromes	Lupus anticoagulant, antiphospholipid
Overlap features such as Raynaud's, myositis, and cardiopulmonary lesions	Anti-RNP
Drug-induced lupus	Anti-histone

Causes of drug-induced lupus

1 Hydralazine
2 Procainamide
3 Phenytoin
4 Isoniazid
5 Penicillamine
6 Methyldopa
7 Propylthiouracil
8 Bleomycin
9 Sulphonamides
10 Minocycline
11 OCP may exacerbate pre-existing SLE.

WHO classification of SLE nephritis

Table 47

Type	Histological appearance
1	Normal
2a	Mesangial deposits
2b	Mesangial hypercellularity
3	Focal segmental nephritis
4	Diffuse proliferative nephritis
5	Membranous nephritis

RHEUMATOLOGY

Pregnancy with SLE

1 No evidence of reduced fertility
2 Pre-existing renal disease may worsen during pregnancy
3 Hypertension more difficult to control
4 Pre-eclampsia difficult to distinguish from renal flare
5 Increased fetal loss in patients with antiphospholipid antibodies
6 Overall no increased risk of fetal abnormalities
7 Antimetabolites contraindicated due to teratogenesis
8 Low-dose prednisolone and azathioprine probably safe
9 Neonatal SLE is a rare complication.

Treatment

1 Sunscreens (photosensitivity)
2 NSAIDs (symptomatic)
3 Chloroquine/hydroxychloroquine (rashes, arthritis, malaise)
4 Corticosteroids for severe flare, low-dose for maintenance
5 Immunosuppressives (azathioprine, methotrexate,
   cyclophosphamide) for severe flare
6 Thalidomide (rash)
7 Dapsone (rash)
8 Plasma exchange in severe cases
9 Anticoagulation for recurrent thromboses
10 Vasodilators (calcium blockers, prostacyclin) for Raynaud's
11 Antihypertensives
12 Anticonvulsants (cerebral lupus).

Antiphospholipid antibody syndrome

1 IgG or IgM antibodies against phospholipids
2 Antibodies may cause a false positive VDRL
3 *In vitro* anticoagulant effect – prolonged APTT which fails to correct
   after addition of normal plasma
4 Predisposes to recurrent thromboses *in vivo*
5 *Clinical features:*
   (a) venous thrombosis:
       (i) DVT
       (ii) major vein thrombosis
       (iii) ocular thrombosis
       (iv) renal vein thrombosis

(v) Budd–Chiari syndrome
(vi) pulmonary hypertension
(b) arterial thrombosis:
(i) limb ischaemia
(ii) stroke/TIA
(iii) MI
(iv) adrenal infarction
(c) recurrent miscarriage
(d) thrombocytopenia
(e) haemolytic anaemia
(f) livedo reticularis
(g) migraine
(h) epilepsy
(i) chorea
(j) myelopathy
(k) heart valve disease
(l) pulmomary hypertension.

Systemic sclerosis (scleroderma)

Systemic sclerosis represents a spectrum of multisystem disorders.

Pre-scleroderma

1 Raynaud's phenomenon
2 Nail-fold capillary changes
3 Circulating antinuclear antibodies (Anti-Scl-70, anticentromere).

Diffuse systemic sclerosis

1 Onset of skin changes within one year of onset of Raynaud's phenomenon
2 Truncal and forearm skin involvement
3 Presence of tendon friction rubs
4 Early and significant incidence of:
(a) interstitial lung disease
(b) oliguric renal failure
(c) diffuse GI disease
(d) myocardial involvement
5 Nail-fold capillary dilatation and capillary dropout
6 Scl-70 antibodies in 30%.

Limited systemic sclerosis

1 Raynaud's phenomenon for years
2 Skin involvement limited to hands, face, feet and forearms, or absent
3 Includes CREST syndrome (calcinosis, Raynaud's, oesophageal involvement, sclerodactyly and telangiectasia)
4 A significant late (10–15 years) incidence of pulmonary hypertension, with or without interstitial lung disease, skin calcinosis, telangiectasia and GI involvement
5 High incidence of anticentromere antibody (70–80%)
6 Dilated nail-fold capillary loops, usually without capillary dropout.

Scleroderma sine scleroderma

1 Raynaud's ±
2 No skin involvement
3 Present with:
    (a) pulmonary fibrosis
    (b) scleroderma renal crisis
    (c) cardiac disease
    (d) GI disease
4 Antinuclear antibodies may be present (Scl-70, centromere, nucleolar).

Overlap syndromes

Features of scleroderma may coexist with those of other autoimmune disorders:
1 SLE
2 RA
3 Dermatomyositis
4 Vasculitis
5 Sjögren's syndrome.

Localised forms

1 Localised morphoea
2 Generalised morphoea
3 Linear scleroderma
4 Coup de sabre.

Clinical features of systemic sclerosis

Musculoskeletal

1 Polyarthralgia
2 Polymyositis.

Skin

1 Raynaud's phenomenon
2 Abnormal nail-fold capillaries
3 Sclerodactyly
4 Telangiectasia
5 Tight smooth waxy pigmented skin
6 Skin ulcers
7 Vitiligo
8 Increased pigmentation
9 Subcutaneous calcification.

Cardiovascular

1 Cardiomyopathy
2 Pericarditis
3 Pericardial effusion
4 Hypertension.

Pulmonary

1 Pulmonary fibrosis
2 Pulmonary hypertension
3 Aspiration pneumonia
4 Bronchiectasis.

Gastointestinal

1 Microstomia and sicca syndrome
2 Dysphagia – poor motility, peptic strictures
3 GORD – low sphincter pressure, hiatus hernia
4 Diverticulae – small bowel, colonic
5 Hypomotility + stasis – can lead to pseudo-obstruction
6 Bacterial overgrowth
7 Malabsorption

8 Pneumatosis intestinalis
9 PBC and chronic active hepatitis.

Renal

1 Progressive renal failure
2 Hypertensive renal crisis.

Neurological

1 Trigeminal neuralgia
2 Autonomic neuropathy.

Raynaud's phenomenon

1 Episodic event characterised by the digits turning white and numb, then cyanosed and finally red and painful (rebound hyperaemia)
2 3–10% of adults affected
3 1% of Raynaud's sufferers have a connective tissue disorder
4 *Causes:*
   (a) idiopathic
   (b) connective tissue disorders
   (c) hypothyroidism
   (d) cervical rib
   (e) cervical spondylosis
   (f) increased plasma viscosity
   (g) syringomyelia
   (h) drugs (beta-blockers, ergot)
   (i) vibrating instruments/tools
5 *Treatment:*
   (a) warmth
   (b) no smoking or beta-blockers
   (c) calcium-channel blockers
   (d) GTN
   (e) ACE inhibitors
   (f) ketanserin (a $5HT_2$ antagonist)
   (g) prostacyclin infusion
   (h) amputation.

Sjögren's syndrome

Sjögren's syndrome may occur in these autoimmune diseases:

1 RA
2 SLE
3 Systemic sclerosis
4 PBC
5 MCTD
6 Mixed cryoglobulinaemia
7 Hashimoto's thyroiditis
8 MS.

Clinical features of primary Sjögren's syndrome

1 Dryness from atrophy of exocrine glands (eyes, mouth, respiratory tract, vagina) (100%)
2 Arthralgia/arthritis (60%)
3 Raynaud's phenomenon (37%)
4 Lymphadenopathy (14%)
5 Vasculitis (11%)
6 RTA type 1 (9%)
7 Liver involvement (7%)
8 Splenomegaly (3%)
9 Peripheral neuropathy (2%)
10 Myositis (1%).

Dermatomyositis and polymyositis

1 Dermatomyositis – idiopathic inflammation of skeletal muscle and cutaneous lesions
2 Polymyositis – similar features without the skin lesions
3 *Cutaneous lesions:*
   (a) heliotrope rash
   (b) nail-fold changes with periungual erythema, cuticular hypertrophy and infarcts
   (c) Gottron's papules (scaly rash on the back of the hands)
   (d) sclerodermatous skin changes with cutaneous and muscular calcification
   (e) Raynaud's disease
4 Proximal muscle weakness
5 Elevated serum levels of muscle enzymes
6 Typical muscle biopsy changes
7 *EMG changes:*
   (a) polyphasic, short, small motor unit potentials

(b) high-frequency repetitive discharges
(c) spontaneous fibrillation
8 Calcification and vasculitis common in the childhood form (more severe)
9 Pulmonary fibrosis, cardiomyopathy and arthropathy may be present
10 Associated with other connective tissue disorders
11 Associated with malignancy in 20% of patients over 50 years of age
12 ANA and anti-Jo-1 antibodies may be present
13 Treatment with steroids and immunosuppressives.

Mixed connective tissue disease (MCTD)

1 Overlap syndrome with features of:
   (a) polymyositis
   (b) systemic sclerosis
   (c) SLE
2 High titre of antibodies to RNP
3 *Clinical features:*
   (a) arthritis (>90%)
   (b) sclerodactyly (90%)
   (c) Raynaud's (80%)
   (d) abnormal oesophageal motility (70%)
   (e) myositis (70%)
   (f) lymphadenopathy
   (g) hepatosplenomegaly
   (h) serositis
   (i) hypergammaglobulinaemia.

Autoantibodies in connective tissue diseases

[See Table 48, opposite]

JUVENILE CHRONIC ARTHRITIS

1 Arthritis in at least one joint for over three months
2 Onset before 16 years
3 Exclusion of other diseases that may cause arthritis.

Pauciarticular (70%)

1 Up to four joints affected in first six months
2 Commonly associated with ANA

Table 48

Antibody	Disease	Specificity	Prevalence
Anti-dsDNA	SLE	High	60%
Anti-Sm	SLE	High	4% Caucasian 30–50% Afro-Caribbean
Anti-Ro	Sjögren's	Low	80%
	SLE		50%
	Congenital neonatal heart block		
Anti-La	Sjögren's	High	50%
	SLE		15%
Anti-RNP	MCTD	Low	90%
	SLE		5%
Anti-Jo-1	Polymyositis	High	25%
	Lung fibrosis		
Anti-Scl-70	Diffuse cutaneous systemic sclerosis	High	25%
Anti-centromere	Limited cutaneous systemic sclerosis	Medium	70%
Anti-cardiolipin	Anti-phospholipid antibody syndrome	Low	
	SLE		
Anti-histones	Drug-induced lupus	Low	60%

3 Strong association with anterior uveitis
4 Good articular prognosis.

Polyarticular (20%)

1 Up to five joints affected in the first six months
2 10% are RF positive (often progress to severe RA).

Systemic – Still's disease (10%)

1 Fever
2 Evanescent, macular, erythematous rash (salmon-pink)
3 Arthritis (usually the systemic features precede arthritis)
4 Organomegaly
5 Lymphadenopathy
6 Can lead to amyloidosis.

REVISED JONES CRITERIA FOR DIAGNOSIS OF ACUTE RHEUMATIC FEVER

Major criteria

1 Carditis
2 Polyarthritis
3 Chorea
4 Erythema marginatum
5 Subcutaneous nodules.

Minor criteria

1 Fever
2 Arthralgia
3 Previous history of rheumatic fever or rheumatic heart disease.

Diagnosis requires two major or one major and two minor, plus evidence of recent streptococcal infection (raised ASO titre or culture of group A streptococci).

DIAGNOSTIC CRITERIA FOR ADULT STILL'S DISEASE

All of these features:
1 Quotidian fever $>39\,°C$
2 Arthralgia/arthritis
3 Negative RF
4 Negative ANA.
Plus two of the following:
1 Leucocytosis $>15 \times 10^9/l$
2 Evanescent macular/maculopapular rash (salmon-pink)
3 Serositis (pleuritic/pericardial)
4 Hepatomegaly
5 Splenomegaly
6 Generalised lymphadenopathy.

RISK FACTORS FOR OA

1 Age

2 Female sex
3 Genetic predisposition
4 Obesity
5 Hypermobility
6 Joint trauma (particularly fractures through the joint)
7 Chondrocalcinosis
8 Infection
9 Hereditary type 2 collagen defects
10 Developmental conditions:
  (a) congenital dislocation of the hip
  (b) Perthes disease
  (c) joint dysplasias
11 Bone disease:
  (a) Paget's disease
  (b) avascular necrosis of bone
  (c) osteopetrosis
12 Endocrine conditions:
  (a) acromegaly
  (b) ochronosis
  (c) haemochromatosis
  (d) Wilson's disease
13 Charcot's joints.

OSTEOPOROSIS – RISK FACTORS AND CAUSES

(see also page 258)

1 Postmenopausal women
2 Elderly
3 Immobility
4 Long-term steroids
5 Lack of oestrogen:
  (a) oophorectomy
  (b) hysterectomy
  (c) obsessional athletes
  (d) early menopause
6 Familial or racial
7 Idiopathic
8 Lack of testosterone in men

  9 RA
10 Cushing's syndrome
11 Thyrotoxicosis
12 Hypopituitarism
13 Anorexia nervosa
14 Starvation
15 Coeliac disease
16 Partial gastrectomy
17 Liver disease
18 Smoking
19 Alcohol
20 Osteogenesis imperfecta
21 Multiple myeloma
22 Metastatic carcinoma
23 Heparin
24 Cytotoxics
25 Anticonvulsants.

VASCULITIS (see also pages 296–297)

Large vessel

Takayasu's arteritis

1 Most commonly presents in females under 40 years
2 Ischaemia or aneurysm formation in the aorta or its branches
3 Often presents with arm claudication and pulseless vessels
4 Diagnosis by angiography.

Giant cell arteritis

1 Typically involves extracranial arteries, leading to ischaemia
2 Diagnosis by temporal artery biopsy (negative biopsy does not exclude diagnosis)
3 *Clinical features:*
  (a) unilateral throbbing headache
  (b) jaw claudication
  (c) amaurosis fugax
  (d) diplopia
  (e) polymyalgia rheumatica symptoms in 50%.

Medium vessel

Polyarteritis nodosa (PAN)

1 Associated with hepatitis B infection
2 American College of Rheumatology criteria for diagnosis of PAN:
  (a) weight loss of > 4 kg
  (b) livedo reticularis
  (c) testicular pain
  (d) myalgia/leg tenderness
  (e) mono/polyneuropathy
  (f) hepatitis Bs Ag positive
  (g) arteriographic abnormality
  (h) positive biopsy.

Kawasaki disease

1 Occurs primarily in children under five years
2 Treatment is with aspirin and high-dose gammaglobulin (reduces mortality from 30% to <1%)
3 *Clinical features:*
  (a) fever for five days or more
  (b) bilateral congestion of conjunctiva without conjunctivitis
  (c) dryness, redness and fissuring of the lips, and inflammation of the oral cavity
  (d) acute non-purulent swelling of the cervical lymph nodes
  (e) skin rash comprising morbilliform, scarlatiniform, urticarious or erythema multiforme-like lesions
  (f) reddening of the palms and soles with oedema, fading to produce desquamation
  (g) coronary artery lesions (aneurysms) in 40% can lead to sudden death, MI or papillary muscle dysfunction.

Small vessel

Churg–Strauss syndrome

1 Asthma
2 Eosinophilia
3 25% cANCA positive; 50% pANCA positive
4 Systemic vasculitis, which may lead to:
  (a) myocarditis

(b) coronary arteritis
(c) pulmonary infiltrate or haemorrhage
(d) stroke
(e) mononeuritis multiplex
(f) GI involvement
(g) renal disease – focal segmental necrotising glomerulonephritis may develop.

Wegener's granulomatosis

1 cANCA positive in > 95%
2 Characterised by upper respiratory tract lesions, pulmonary disease and glomerulonephritis
3 *Clinical features:*
  (a) upper respiratory tract (90%):
    (i) epistaxis
    (ii) purulent nasal discharge
    (iii) sinusitis
    (iv) destruction of nasal septum
  (b) lower respiratory tract (90%):
    (i) pulmonary infiltrates
    (ii) pulmonary haemorrhage
  (c) kidney:
    (i) proteinuria
    (ii) haematuria
    (iii) focal necrotising GN
    (iv) renal failure
  (d) other features:
    (i) polyarthralgia
    (ii) myalgia
    (iii) vasculitic rash
    (iv) nail-fold infarcts
    (v) pericarditis
    (vi) arrhythmias
    (vii) scleritis
    (viii) uveitis
    (ix) proptosis (retro-orbital granuloma formation)
    (x) mononeuritis multiplex.

Microscopic polyangiitis

1 Vasculitis affects single organ or multisystems
2 pANCA positive
3 *Clinical features:*
  (a) kidney (almost 100%):
    (i) glomerulonephritis
    (ii) microscopic haematuria
  (b) lung:
    (i) pulmonary haemorrhage
    (ii) pleurisy
    (iii) pleural effusions
  (c) other features:
    (i) purpuric rash
    (ii) arthralgia
    (iii) mononeuritis multiplex
    (iv) GI symptoms
    (v) pericarditis
    (vi) arrhythmias.

Henoch–Schönlein purpura

1 Most common systemic vasculitis in children
2 IgA deposited in the skin and kidney
3 Preceded by upper respiratory tract infection in 90%
4 *Clinical features:*
  (a) purpuric rash (100%) – lower limbs and buttocks
  (b) arthralgia
  (c) glomerulonephritis
  (d) GI bleeding
  (e) intussusception.

Polymyalgia rheumatica (PMR)

1 Most common in patients aged 60–70 years
2 One-third of patients are under 60 years
3 25% have giant cell arteritis
4 Raised ESR and ALP (30%)
5 Symptoms and ESR respond rapidly to steroids
6 *Clinical features* (often sudden onset):
  (a) proximal muscle weakness, worse in the morning

    (b) malaise
    (c) weight loss
    (d) joint pain
    (e) depression
    (f) symptoms of giant cell arteritis (see above).

ANTI-NEUTROPHIL CYTOPLASMIC ANTIBODY (ANCA)

[See Table 49, opposite]

FAMILIAL MEDITERRANEAN FEVER

1 Polyserositis
2 Affects Arabs, Jews, Armenians and Turks
3 *Clinical features:*
    (a) abdominal pain from peritonitis
    (b) vomiting
    (c) constipation
    (d) pyrexia
    (e) pleurisy
    (f) large-joint arthritis
    (g) rash
    (h) cutaneous vasculitis
    (i) myalgia
    (j) episcleritis
    (k) headaches
    (l) pericarditis
    (m) splenomegaly
4 Often develop amyloidosis
5 Diagnosed using intravenous metraminole
6 Treated with long-term colchicine.

CRYOGLOBULINAEMIA

1 Immunoglobulins that reversibly precipitate in the cold ($< 4\,°C$)

Table 49

Auto-antibody	Distribution of staining	Antigen	Diseases
cANCA	Cytoplasm	Proteinase 3(PR3)	Wegener's granulomatosis
pANCA	Perinuclear	Myeloperoxidase (MPO)	Microscopic polyangiitis
			Idiopathic GN
pANCA	Perinuclear	Non-specific subset, binding:	SLE
		Elastase	MCTD
		Lactoferrin	UC
		Lysozyme	RTA
			CFA
			CAH

2 *Types:*
   [See Table 50, opposite]
3 *Clinical features:*
   (a) purpura
   (b) arthralgia
   (c) leg ulcers
   (d) Raynaud's
   (e) abdominal pain
   (f) Sjögren's syndrome
   (g) sensorimotor peripheral neuropathy
   (h) liver disease
   (i) renal disease (mesangiocapillary nephritis)
4 Treat with alpha-interferon if hepatitis C positive.

FIBROMYALGIA

Symptoms

1 Pain:
   (a) predominantly neck and back (may be all over)
   (b) aggravated by stress, cold, activity
2 Generalised morning stiffness
3 Paraesthesiae of hands and feet
4 Fatiguability
5 Non-restorative sleep
6 Headache
7 Diffuse abdominal pain and variable bowel habit
8 Urinary frequency
9 Dysmenorrhoea.

Signs

1 Discordance between symptoms, disability and objective findings
2 No objective weakness, synovitis or neurological abnormality
3 Multiple hyperalgesic sites
4 Pronounced tenderness to rolling the mid trapezius skin fold
5 Cutaneous hyperaemia after palpation of tender sites
6 Negative control sites.

Table 50

	Type 1	Type 2	Type 3
Composition	Monoclonal immunoglobulin, usually IgM or IgG	Monoclonal IgM RF + polyclonal IgG	Polyclonal IgM RF + polyclonal IgG
Disease associations	Myeloma Waldenstrom's macroglobulinaemia Lymphoproliferative disease	Bacterial endocarditis Hep C Hep B EBV CMV	Lyme disease Syphilis Malaria SLE RA Sjögren's syndrome Systemic sclerosis Mixed essential cryoglobulinaemia

MALIGNANT TUMOURS OF BONE

[See Table 51, opposite]

CAUSES OF AVASCULAR NECROSIS OF BONE

1 Corticosteroids/Cushing's
2 Fractured neck of femur
3 Severe OA/RA
4 Sickle cell disease
5 Heparin therapy
6 SLE
7 Pregnancy
8 Chronic exposure to raised barometric pressure (divers)
9 Alcohol
10 Diabetes
11 Obesity
12 Polycythaemia rubra vera
13 Neuropathic joint
14 Bacterial endocarditis
15 Perthes disease
16 Thiemann's disease (AD, affects small joints of the hands and feet).

CAUSES OF CHARCOT'S JOINTS

1 Neurosyphilis
2 Syringomyelia
3 Myelomeningocele
4 Leprosy
5 Diabetes
6 Charcot–Marie–Tooth disease.

RHEUMATOLOGICAL DISEASES ASSOCIATED WITH MALIGNANCY

1 Dermatomyositis – carcinoma

Table 51

Tumour	Age	Common sites	Behaviour	Treatment and prognosis
Osteosarcoma	Young adults	Long bones, esp. distal femur and proximal tibia	Rapid growth, pain and swelling, lung metastases	Surgery and chemotherapy 40% cure rate
Chondrosarcoma	35–60 years	Pelvis, ribs, spine, long bones	Slow enlargement, eventual vascular invasion	Surgery 75% cure rate
Fibrosarcoma Malignant fibrous histiocytoma	Any age, peak 30–40	Femur, tibia, humerus, pelvis	Local growth, vascular invasion	Surgery 40% cure rate
Ewing's sarcoma	Children and teenagers	Long bones, pelvis and ribs	Widespread metastases	Chemotherapy 10% cure rate

2 Scleroderma – adenocarcinoma
3 Primary Sjögren's syndrome – lymphoma
4 RA – lymphoma, myeloma.

CAUSES OF A VERY HIGH ESR (>100 mm/hour)

1 Multiple myeloma
2 Giant cell arteritis/PMR
3 Sepsis
4 Occult malignancy
5 SLE.

SIDE-EFFECTS OF DRUGS USED IN RHEUMATOLOGY

NSAIDs

Gastrointestinal

1 Dyspepsia + gastritis
2 GU/DU
3 Diarrhoea
4 Hepatitis.

CNS

1 Headache and dizziness
2 Tinnitus
3 Aseptic meningitis
4 Confusion.

Cardiovascular

1 Oedema
2 Hypertension
3 Heart failure.

Pulmonary

1 Asthma
2 Pneumonitis.

Blood

1 Neutropenia
2 Thrombocytopenia
3 Aplastic anaemia
4 Haemolytic anaemia.

Renal

1 ARF
2 Haematuria
3 Nephrotic syndrome
4 Papillary necrosis
5 Interstitial nephritis.

Skin

1 Erythema multiforme
2 Fixed drug eruption.

Anti-rheumatoid drugs

Hydroxychloroquine

1 Pruritic skin rash
2 Pigmentation
3 Maculopathy
4 Leucopenia.

Gold

1 Dermatitis (30%)
2 Stomatitis
3 Proteinuria
4 Thrombocytopenia
5 Leucopenia
6 Aplastic anaemia
7 Diarrhoea.

Penicillamine

1 Maculopapular rash

2 Nausea
3 Loss of taste sensation
4 Mouth ulcers
5 Proteinura
6 Nephrotic syndrome
7 Drug-induced lupus
8 Myasthenia gravis
9 Pemphigus
10 Goodpasture's syndrome
11 Thrombocytopenia
12 Pancytopenia.

Sulfasalazine

1 Nausea
2 Skin rashes
3 Allergic reactions
4 Hepatitis
5 Pulmonary eosinophilia
6 Macrocytosis
7 Haemolytic anaemia
8 Pancytopenia
9 Oligospermia (reversible).

Methotrexate

1 Hepatic fibrosis
2 Blood dyscrasias.

Cyclophosphamide

1 Haemorrhagic cystitis
2 Pancytopenia.

Index